Social policy towards 2000

Governments in all advanced industrial societies are involved in an endless struggle to 'square the welfare circle'. Demand for public services rises due to demographic, social and labour market factors, while government ability to finance this demand is constrained by economic and, at times, ideological factors.

The contributors to this book, all well-known academics in the social policy field, analyse the factors that have accounted for the rise in public demand for social welfare in the United Kingdom. They investigate the country's ability and willingness to provide the necessary funds for good quality service during the 1990s and beyond. *Social Policy Towards 2000* documents the economic and social policy changes of the Thatcher years and looks at the current situation in relation to employment, social security, education, health, housing and the personal social services. The contributors compare the proposals of the three main political parties for the welfare system in the years up to 2000 and present a prospective analysis of the future of welfare in the UK. Their general conclusion is that if present policy trends continue, the welfare state in Britain will be scaled down to a residual form by the year 2000 or soon after.

An important contribution to the debate on 'squaring the welfare circle', *Social Policy Towards 2000* will be of special value to students, lecturers and professionals in social policy, social work, sociology and political science.

Vic George is Professor of Social Policy and Social Work at the University of Kent. **Stewart Miller** is Lecturer in Social Policy at the University of Kent.

Social policy towards 2000

Squaring the welfare circle

Edited by Vic George
and Stewart Miller

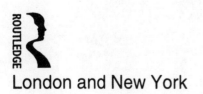

London and New York

First published 1994
by Routledge
11 New Fetter Lane, London EC4P 4EE

Simultaneously published in the USA and Canada
by Routledge
29 West 35th Street, New York, NY 10001

Typeset in Baskerville by
NWL Editorial Services, Langport, Somerset
Printed and bound in Great Britain by
Mackays of Chatham PLC, Chatham, Kent

British Library Cataloguing in Publication Data
A catalogue record for this book is available from the
British Library

Library of Congress Cataloging in Publication Data
Social policy towards 2000: squaring the welfare
circle/edited by Vic George and Stewart Miller.
p. cm.
Includes bibliographical references and index.
1. Great Britain – Social policy – 1979– . 2. Public
welfare – Great Britain. I. George, Victor. II. Miller,
Stewart, 1946– .
HN390.S64 1993   93–15045
361.6'1'0941 – dc20   CIP

ISBN 0–415–08706–6
     0–415–08707–4 (pbk)

Contents

Tables

Contributors

The editors and contributors are all present or former members of the Social Science Faculty of the University of Kent at Canterbury (UKC).

John Baldock is a Senior Lecturer in Social Policy at UKC. He is the author of articles and reports on social care, notably on innovation in social care in Europe.

Hartley Dean is a Senior Lecturer in Social Policy at Luton College of Higher Education. He is the author of *Social Security and Social Control* (Routledge 1991).

Vic George is Professor of Social Policy and Social Work at UKC. He has written numerous books on social policy, on social security and on poverty, including *Wealth, Poverty and Starvation* (Wheatsheaf 1988).

Sean Glynn is a Senior Lecturer in Economic and Social History at UKC. He has written books and articles on employment and unemployment, including *No Alternative? Unemployment in Britain* (Faber 1991).

Nick Manning is a Reader in Social Policy at UKC. He has written extensively on comparative social policy and on health questions, including *The Therapeutic Community Movement* (Routledge 1989).

Stewart Miller is Lecturer in Social Policy at UKC. He has written on social problems and on citizenship.

Peter Taylor-Gooby is Professor of Social Policy at UKC. He has published many articles and several books on the welfare state, including *Public Opinion, Ideology and State Welfare* (Routledge and Kegan Paul 1985).

Clare Ungerson is a Professor of Social Policy at Southampton University. She has published books and other pieces on housing, women and informal care, including *Policy is Personal* (Tavistock 1987).

Introduction

Most books in social policy have so far adopted either a historical, retrospective or contemporary, current approach to the study of social policy issues. In recent years, there has been a growing awareness that the current and historical approaches must be complemented with the prospective approach, which attempts to look at possible social policy developments in the near future (Ermisch 1990; Manning and Page 1992). This book attempts to give due emphasis to this new prospective approach. It is concerned with the development of social policy towards the new century in the light of economic, social, demographic and political trends of the 1980s and early 1990s.

The book also departs from the tradition of social policy studies in a second important way. It systematically analyses and compares the social policy proposals of Britain's three main political parties – Conservative, Labour, and Liberal Democrat – at the beginning of the 1990s and the implications of these proposals for the development of social policy for the rest of the decade. The three party political positions are examined in the context of current and future trends in the economy, in demography, in social change and in public attitudes towards the welfare state.

The overarching framework within which the debates in all the chapters are conducted centres on what we have called 'the squaring of the welfare circle'. We use the term to convey the continual and intensifying struggle of governments in all advanced industrial societies to preserve an equilibrium between (a) meeting the constantly rising need and demand for welfare provision and (b) meeting simultaneous demands for limiting public expenditure, while maintaining electoral acceptability. A complex web of interacting economic, political, social and demographic factors determines the ways in which governments attempt to bridge the gap between public revenues and public policy provisions – to square the welfare circle. The mathematical difficulty of finding the square that matches the area of a given circle or vice versa is proverbial, as is the attempt to square the welfare circle – to meet social service demand with sufficient social service finance.

Interestingly enough, this concern with squaring the welfare circle became a feature of party political activity from the mid-1970s onwards. The creators of the post-war welfare state had fewer such concerns. They were confident that the state possessed enough resources to meet public social needs in a universalist framework of provision. It was not until the mid-1970s that political parties in this country began to express doubts about the economic viability of the Beveridgean–Keynesian universalist welfare state. Out of these doubts emerged the concept, which we have called 'the affordable welfare state', that has come to command party political support today and which influences substantially party political approaches to social policy issues. This historical development from the universalist to the affordable welfare state is the subject of Chapter 1.

It was Prime Minister Margaret Thatcher who first attempted to implement this new version of the welfare state. Chapter 2 thus examines the economic and social policy changes of the 1980s. It shows that the economic record of the Thatcher years was more of a mirage than a miracle. While economic productivity improved, the rate of economic growth for the decade was no better than that of previous decades as a result of the decline in the manufacturing sector and the soaring rates of unemployment. The social policy changes of the decade were profound, and are destined to have a long-lasting impact. In housing, public expenditure was cut drastically through the sale of council housing; in health and education, public expenditure remained fairly static, while in social security it rose as a result of the growing number of claimants. It is the new methods of providing and administering the services that are likely to have a long-lasting impact: the emphasis on fixed annual budgets, on privatisation, on contracting out and on internal markets. These have changed considerably our perception of what is to be expected of the social services; the balance between need and funding as determinants of provision has shifted towards the latter, the role of which has become much more explicit.

Trends in the economy, in demography and in society seem likely to intensify the conflicts and dilemmas involved in squaring the welfare circle during the 1990s. Although difficult to predict accurately, it is generally accepted that rates of economic growth and of unemployment will show little or no improvement on those of the 1980s. On the other side of the equation, demographic and social trends will increase demand for social services. When these two are considered in the light of party political competition to offer low-tax policies for electoral gain, the prospects for policy to meet social needs are not encouraging. All these issues are the concern of Chapter 3.

Full employment is central to the provision of an adequately funded welfare state, as Glynn shows in Chapter 4. The proceeds of full employment include both individual welfare resources for the employed and the state revenues that finance government services. It also reduces expenditure on benefits for the un-employed. Glynn also argues that, while there are substantial differences between the main parties on employment policy, all three have been converted to, or at least have accepted as inevitable, a balance of economic priorities which emphasises the achievement of low inflation, even at the cost of tolerating high levels of unemployment. Glynn's conclusion that rates of economic growth and unemployment will not improve in the 1990s and will have adverse implications for social welfare echoes our own argument in Chapter 3.

Social security constitutes the largest item of government expenditure. Dean's discussion in Chapter 5 shows that Conservative policies in this area will continue to emphasise the selective targeting of benefits; the Labour Party, although committed to universalism in the long term, shows extreme caution in its policies for the 1990s; while the Liberal Democrats, more radically, propose the merging of benefit and taxation systems and the gradual introduction of a minimum income guarantee scheme. Demographic and social changes have brought to the fore new groups of the poor, notably the unemployed and lone-parent families. Dean's conclusion is that, despite the fact that social security expenditure will remain high, the level of benefits will not improve and the risk of poverty will remain high for the rest of the decade.

All three parties stress the importance of education, which they all see both as a form of human capital investment and a means of facilitating individual advancement and development. But they differ in the relative emphasis they give to these functions of education, although none delve very deeply into the conflicts between them in terms of policy goals. Taylor-Gooby, in Chapter 6, points to a number of significant differences between the parties on the best way of administering education, on the role of parents and professionals, on the relationship between local and central government, on the size of the private sector and on what is an adequate level of funding for the state sector. Recent educational reforms which give prominence to choice and participation at the expense of the social considerations of class, gender and race inequalities seem likely to dominate debates in the 1990s.

Health, with its traditions of professional autonomy and influence, is perhaps the area where the shift towards the ubiquitous and explicit dominance of resource considerations has attracted most public attention. In Chapter 7, Manning examines the significance of demographic, social, political, economic and technological factors on health care and finds that they will continue to exert upward demand pressures in the future. None of the political parties take sufficient account of this in their funding proposals. As in education, so too in health care: the parties differ on the best ways of administering the service and particularly on the role of internal markets in social service provision. Manning draws attention to the ideological nature of currently dominant views of what a country can afford to spend on social services.

The personal social services have always been the Cinderella of social policy, grossly underfunded and never featuring prominently in the manifestos or campaigns of any of the parties. It has never been the policy of any government or party to make universal provision in this area. For all the recent rhetoric on the value of community care and all the social and demographic evidence pointing to increasing need and increasing demand, there is no effective commitment of the resources necessary to square this particular circle. As Baldock points out in Chapter 8, policy developments in the personal social services 'are almost always reactive and spasmodic'. Could it be that the reason for this is the absence of politically strong lobbies, either on the professional or the consumer side?

Ungerson's account of the housing question in the 1980s in Chapter 9 shows quite clearly how much has changed in this area of policy. The intense emphasis on owner occupation, the sale of council housing and the continuing decline of the privately rented sector has meant not only a marked reduction in public expenditure on housing but also a new set of housing problems: mortgage arrears and evictions on an unprecedented scale and a rise in homelessness, as well as neglect and disrepair across all types of housing tenure. All parties are united in support of owner occupation; what divides them is the relative size and role of the social housing sector, although even here they agree on the need for tenant participation in day-to-day management. They all recognise the importance of housing in the economy, but differ in their degree of caution in using this sector to stimulate economic activity. Ungerson rightly observes that in the field of housing there are many circles to be squared.

Chapter 10 briefly summarises the agreements and disagreements of the parties across the range of social policies. It then explores the basic assumptions of social politics today, which are inexorably leading Britain towards a residual welfare state. It ends by suggesting that these are not the only assumptions on which social politics can be based towards and through the turn of the century, and that alternative visions of welfare remain viable. These alternatives include something much more like a citizens' welfare state: a participatory welfare system, mixed in form but universalist in rights.

Chapter 1

Squaring the welfare circle

Vic George and Stewart Miller

Governments in all advanced industrial societies today are engaged in an intensifying struggle: first, to meet the increasing public demand for high quality welfare provision; second, to meet the simultaneous public demand for limiting levels of taxation; third, to maintain and raise rates of economic growth; and fourth, to maintain and improve their electoral chances. It is this difficult balancing act that the phrase 'squaring the welfare circle' describes. The welfare circle is public service provision and the welfare square is public service finance. Mathematicians today take the thoroughly modern view that no formula can be found for perfectly squaring the physical circle and that this is a fact of life with which we must all live. It is a conclusion that social scientists pondering over ways of squaring the welfare circle may find slightly disheartening, even though it should not prevent them from looking for ways that get pretty close to it.

This chapter examines how the debate on squaring the welfare circle has evolved in Britain, bearing in mind that this was not a dominant preoccupation among either politicians or social scientists in the 1940s when the Labour government reforms created the post-war welfare state. Since this is not merely a British dilemma, references are made to how some other industrial societies have tried to cope with the problem.

The post-war welfare state in Britain was based on very considerable political consensus which reflected agreement between the major political parties in three main areas. First, the government had both the capacity and the duty to manage the economy in such a way as to increase economic growth and to maintain full employment. Second, the government could and should engage in a wide variety of interventions designed to improve the quality of life. Third, the government had both the resources and the responsibility to provide a range of universalist social services available to all, free at the point of use, as a substantial contribution to ensuring a basic and rising standard of living for all its citizens. An open but regulated market and a coherent package of social provision complemented each other to the benefit of both economic growth and social protection. It was a political consensus that reflected both the public mood and the nature of British society of that time.

It was this blend of Keynesian economics and Beveridgean social concern that gave the welfare state its strong political legitimacy and popular appeal. This is not to suggest that there were no party political differences in the details of policy programmes or that there were no dissenting voices from both the left and the right. It is the dissent from the right, however, that concerns us most here, because it was this that eventually became a mainstream critique of the universalist welfare state. At the theoretical level, before it was even realised, Hayek denounced the universalist welfare state as 'the road to serfdom', the route away from both economic growth and personal freedom. Substantial central government planning and provision, he asserted, necessarily result in political dictatorship as they concentrate too much power in the hands of the government and render its leaders increasingly intolerant of opposing groups. Democratic central planning on a large scale was, to him, a contradiction in terms. Only 'a policy of freedom for the individual' could reverse the trend towards collectivism and authoritarianism that was so evident in Europe in the 1930s and 1940s (Hayek 1944: 178). At the political and industrial level, there were also misgivings about the implications of universal social provision on the economy. No less a figure than Winston Churchill, influenced by Hayek's thesis, warned his wartime cabinet colleagues against the financial burden of the Beveridge Report proposals and the 'false hopes and visions of Utopia and Eldorado' engendered by the report (Churchill, in Jones *et al.* 1978: 48). A group of Conservative MPs signed a letter in 1944 protesting against the collectivist trend of government legislation: 'Bill after Bill is being introduced, or envisaged, which involves compulsion and loss of personal Freedom' (Greenleaf 1983: 310). Similarly, the President of the Federation of British Industries urged the Labour government in 1947 'not to rush their programme and to place production and prosperity above party plans and policies' (Rogow and Shore 1955: 13).

Opposition to the universalist welfare state became more conceptual and policy specific during the late 1950s and 1960s. A great deal of this critical literature emerged from the Institute of Economic Affairs. One of its earliest papers by Lees in 1961 laid out many of the arguments that would appear in later literature from the new right. Concentrating on the NHS, Lees argued that medical care was 'not markedly different' from the goods that people bought in the private market and there was, therefore, no good reason why it should not be provided by the private market. Indeed, it was the best way to open the NHS to 'consumer choice', to make it more efficient and rid it of its fundamental weaknesses – 'the dominance of political decisions, the absence of built-in forces making for improvement and the removal of the test of the market' (Lees 1961: 78).

Conservative politicians with ministerial experience began in the 1960s to question the government's expanding role in economic and social affairs. Enoch Powell, with the experience of an ex-Minister of Health, came to the conclusion that the method of funding the NHS was at the bottom of many of the ills of the service. It 'endows everyone providing as well as using it with a vested interest in denigrating it' in an effort to extract even more funds from the central government (Powell 1966: 16). A couple of years later he widened his attack on the welfare state by putting the blame for the economic problems of the country substantially on the rise in public expenditure. 'On any view, the margin by which public expenditure has overshot the growth of the national income is the *major cause* of the disastrous financial events of the last four years, which still pursue us: internal inflation, external devaluation, and foreign indebtedness' (Powell 1970: 111). Thus by the early 1970s the anti-welfare state lobby was well established in Britain even though it commanded very little academic, political or public support. The material base for the spread of new right ideas was still unfavourable. Ideas do not take hold in a socio-economic vacuum: social and economic conditions must be such as to lend credence to new ideas before they are widely accepted, taken on board by governments and generally replace previous orthodoxies. Before we discuss these changes, it is useful to look briefly at the left-wing critique of the welfare state during this period.

The discovery that the extensive – and expensive – welfare system established under the post-war settlement had not substantially reduced wealth and income inequalities (Titmuss 1962) and had not even abolished subsistence poverty (Abel-Smith and Townsend 1965) was at once a blow to optimists of the left and a cause of tension among those of differing views on the state's ability to deal effectively with these problems in a capitalist society. Fabian socialists remained inherently optimistic about the potential of capitalism for reform and gradual improvement while many Marxists denied such potential and maintained their suspicion that post-war reform was fundamentally a smokescreen and a sop (Miliband 1969). Whatever the misgivings, however, the critical left argued not for the reduction but for the expansion of the welfare state as well as for more vertically redistributive forms of taxation.

These criticisms from the right and left remained marginal until material changes in society in general and in people's living standards in particular became strong enough to enable a more widespread acceptance of new ideas. Unfortunately for the left, material changes favoured the ideas of the right. Three main societal changes had been gradually taking place throughout the 1950s and 1960s which separately and together began to present a serious challenge to the universalist social service welfare state. The first sprang from the increasing economic affluence that the country experienced through these two decades. Rising standards of living – increasingly taken for granted – meant rising aspirations in both the economic and social fields. People formed expectations of the social services that outstripped service performance. They began to draw comparisons between the 'quality of service' they received in the private market and that received when using the social services – and they found these services wanting, both in the physical standards they experienced and in the way they were treated by professionals providing the services. The second main trend was the decline in the relative economic performance of the country. Rates of economic growth, of profitability and of investment were falling, while rates of unemployment and inflation were gradually rising, and rates of taxation inevitably moved upwards to provide the funds for the welfare state. Thus rising public aspirations and hence demands on the public services were accompanied by enhanced economic difficulties in the way of meeting them. Third, the diversification of the occupational structure meant that the country was no longer merely a two- or three-class society. Conflicts of economic interest increasingly manifested themselves among the various subgroups making up the various classes. Both taxation rates and social policy provision affected these various subgroups differently, with the result that the support of some of them for the universalist welfare state weakened considerably. All these changes produced a climate that was favourable for the flourishing of the new right ideology which had hitherto remained dormant. There was, however, no inevitability about this. If the left had modified its policies to take account of the societal changes and attitudes towards welfare, it might have been able to preserve the long-standing political consensus on the welfare state.

Indeed, by the early 1970s major political figures in the Labour Party were beginning to voice their concerns on how to square the welfare circle. Their commitment to the universal welfare state remained as strong as ever, but their faith in the ability of governments to square the welfare circle was shaken by their experience as ministers in the Labour governments of the 1960s.

It was Crosland who first acknowledged the unenviable task of governments trying to finance expanding welfare services during periods of low economic growth. By 1969, the United Kingdom ranked third in the OECD – after the Netherlands and Sweden – in terms of public expenditure as a proportion of GDP. Writing in the very early 1970s, he warned of the inflationary dangers involved in financing expanding public services through constantly rising rates of taxation. Only increased rates of economic growth could sustain high levels of public expenditure and preserve public support for the welfare state. Moreover, high rates of economic growth were indispensable to the creation of a socialist society. They were not sufficient in themselves but, he argued, 'in a democracy low or zero growth wholly excludes the possibility' (Crosland 1974: 74). With disarming honesty, he admitted that the Labour Party did not have 'some panacea for crisis-free growth which was mysteriously hidden from both the previous Labour and the present Tory Governments' (1974: 58). Two years later, and now in government, he made his now famous statement that 'The party is over' (Crosland 1982: 295). Unless and until rates of economic growth improved, the harsh reality was that growth in public expenditure was impossible. This call to financial prudence gradually became part of Labour government thinking so that the two main parties in the country began to converge on this issue in later years.

It was within this new economic and political climate that social scientists of the right and left began to develop their new pessimistic scenarios of the future of the welfare state. Two seminal articles of 1975 sketched out elements which were to be central to the new right account of the welfare state crisis in Britain. Both reached the same conclusion: that the welfare state was expected to perform so many functions and to provide so many services that it could not cope, and could not carry on any longer in such a condition. The first article, by Samuel Brittan, saw the causes of this crisis in the competitive nature of democratic systems. In a parliamentary democracy, competing interest groups exert pressure on political parties which vie with each other for election and re-election, with the result that there is 'a systemic upward bias to expectations' (Brittan 1975: 141). Thus a continuous expansion of government services and functions takes place without enough thought being given to the ill consequences of this process.

Anthony King, in the other key article, presented the 'overload' of government as the result of structural factors related to the increased industrialisation, urbanisation, and indeed internationalisation, of British society. What happens at work, for example, has implications for people's lives at home, in the market-place and elsewhere. Urbanisation creates both possibilities and problems which affect people's lives in many diverse and complex ways. Thus governments which decide to act in one area find themselves forced by this interaction to enter others too. But the more governments take on, the less they can deliver, for so many problems turn out to be beyond their capacity. They do not possess the resources or the knowledge to tackle many of the problems forced on them. One of the possible consequences of this 'overloading' of governments was public loss of faith in parliamentary democracy. As King put it:

> Although no-one has produced a plausible scenario for the collapse of the British system of government the fact that people are talking about the possibility at all is in itself significant, and certainly we seem likely in the mid or late 1970s to face the sort of 'crisis of the regime' that Britain has not known since 1832, possibly not since the seventeenth century.
>
> (King 1975: 294–5)

Thus for both Brittan and King the crisis was primarily a political issue of credibility and legitimation not only for individual governments but for the democratic system itself. The only solution was a reduction in government activities – and promises – but both Brittan and King saw this as being very difficult to bring about because of the systemic nature of the causes of crisis. Their proposals, therefore, were limited to appeals to the politicians, to the mass media and to others to scale down the demands made on governments.

It was, however, the writings of economists consciously identifying themselves with the economic liberal tradition that proved more immediately telling for the future development of the welfare state. In the mid-1970s, Bacon and Eltis placed the blame – as did Powell before them – for what was to them the crucial decline of the manufacturing sector of the British economy, firmly and squarely on the rise in public expenditure and public employment. The de-industrialisation thesis, as it came to be known, proved very influential because its promotion almost coincided with the recession of the late 1970s. It was a simplistic and largely erroneous explanation for a complex problem but it rang true to those who were anxious to reduce public expenditure on political, industrial and other grounds. Public expenditure, it was argued, led to a reduction of profits and investment and to a rise in wages and taxes; it tipped the balance of industrial relations in favour of the trade unions; and it undermined work and savings incentives. Above all, 'successive governments have allowed large numbers of workers to move out of industry and into various service occupations' where they mostly consume but do not produce (Bacon and Eltis 1976: 221). Britain's public sector expanded at the expense of the manufacturing sector and a radical change was needed to reverse the downward spiral in the country's fortunes: reduce the level of public expenditure and public employment and, at a stroke, make more funds and labour available for deployment in the manufacturing sector. This was clearly an attractive analysis for rightist politicians seeking to distance themselves not only from Labour but from the whole 'disastrous' history of post-war public sector growth. As early as 1975, Margaret Thatcher, the new leader of the Conservative Party, had stressed that the public sector was in competition with the private not only for revenue and capital but also for labour: 'Every man switched away from industry and into Government will reduce the productive sector and increase the burden on it at the same time' (Cooke 1989: 12).

Thus the right-wing critique of the welfare state came to combine the economic with the political. Its message was that the political and economic crisis of the country could be solved through a reduction in public expenditure, public employment and public provision. The public services were seen as a drain on the political and economic strength of the country. A reversal of post-war welfare expansionism would at once reduce personal reliance on the state; cut taxes; undermine the strength of the trade unions and thus their ability to obtain unrealistic wage rises; and improve profitability, growth rates and general economic prosperity. The welfare circle would be squared. There would be short-term difficulties and problems but in the longer term the country would learn to live within its means and prosper. Although these ideas had been expressed before, they rang more true now for they appeared to make more sense of economic realities. They made more sense of Friedman's dictum 25 years earlier that 'one cannot be both an egalitarian and a liberal' (Friedman 1962: 195).

Writing at the same time as the overload theorists, O'Connor and Habermas provided a Marxian critique of advanced welfare capitalism. Fundamentally, their argument was that the state in capitalist societies was forced to provide two types of services: those which made the capitalist system more efficient and profitable – education, roads, research, and so on – and those which improved the political acceptability of the system among the masses – social security benefits, and the like. Both types were necessary to the survival of the capitalist system. In carrying out these services, however, the state had to resort to increased spending which it found more and more difficult to finance, since it was not the state itself but the capitalist class which was benefiting directly from the increased profitability resulting from these expensive interventions. In O'Connor's terms, the 'fiscal crisis' of the state was a structural phenomenon inherent in all welfare capitalist societies. It could not be solved within the capitalist institutional order: if the state reduced its expenditure it would make the system either less profitable or less politically acceptable or both. In his opinion, 'the only lasting solution to the crisis is socialism' (O'Connor 1973: 221). Only the socialisation of the means of production could solve the fiscal crisis because the state would then collect the profits to pay for its services. Habermas adopted a similar line but was less inclined to dismiss the ability of governments to cope somehow with their deep-rooted problems. The capitalist state would attempt to resolve the crisis through a variety of *ad hoc* measures – some reductions in public expenditure, promotion of private services, increased resort to authoritarian measures, and so on (Habermas 1975: 75). In the final analysis, however, Habermas concluded that the welfare circle could not be squared within a capitalist welfare society, because public pressure for greater participation in and consumption of public services was irreversible in democratic societies.

Thus the Marxist 'state contradiction' and the right-wing 'overloading' theories agreed on the basic features of the fiscal and legitimation crisis but disagreed on its causes and remedies. Moreover, they were both very pessimistic that a solution to the crisis was possible. It was left to writers of the centre to strike a more balanced, or perhaps less alarmist, note. Such writers acknowledged that welfare states in all advanced capitalist societies faced problems of legitimacy but asserted that these did not constitute an overloading or a fiscal or legitimation crisis. Their main focus of concern was the relationship between the economy and public service provision. So long as rates of economic growth were healthy enough to finance growing demands for public provision, as was the case in the 1950s and 1960s, all was well. When this was not possible, as was the case in the late 1970s when the economic recession engulfed the whole world, governments had a difficult task in rationing resources. Writing in 1979, Rose and Peters expressed this well when they proclaimed that 'the greatest challenge facing the governors of every western country today is the maintenance of political authority in the face of economic difficulties' (Rose and Peters 1979: 6). They hastened to add, however, that 'to suggest that a country with economic difficulties could become ungovernable is literally to talk nonsense' (1979: 6). Governments had the difficult task of finding the right balance between public services provision and taxation rates. The public were right to expect services as of right as well as tolerable taxation rates. It was the duty of governments to find the politically acceptable balance between the two. It was difficult but both necessary and possible. Thus references to 'legitimation crisis' and 'ungovernability' were exaggerations and governments could, with prudence and judicious *adhoc*ery, steer their way through the troubled waters. Despite this calmer analysis, it was the concepts of 'overloading' and 'fiscal crisis' that seemed to have exerted more influence on party political attitudes towards the welfare state in Britain at this time.

During the late 1970s, Britain was in the unenviable position of having, on one hand, one of the highest rates of public expenditure and direct taxation and, on the other, one of the lowest rates of economic growth among OECD countries. The only way the Callaghan government could square the welfare circle was through a combination of borrowing from the IMF and a reduction of public expenditure. It was in anticipation of this deal with the IMF that Callaghan, in his speech as Prime Minister to his party conference in 1976, was at pains to distance himself from earlier brands of economic and fiscal policies.

> For too long, perhaps ever since the war, we postponed facing up to fundamental choices and fundamental changes in our society and in our economy. . . . We used to think that you could spend your way out of a recession and increase employment by cutting taxes and boosting government spending. I tell you in all candour that the option no longer exists, and that in so far as it ever did exist, it only worked on each occasion since the war by injecting a bigger dose of inflation into the economy followed by a higher level of unemployment as the next step.
>
> (Parsons 1982: 426)

This was a reiteration and an extension of the Crosland thesis that neither increased taxation nor increased borrowing could for long sustain high rates of public expenditure without damaging the economy.

It was not surprising, therefore, that by the late 1970s the Conservative Party was ready to abandon the Keynesian–Beveridgean post-war settlement. Margaret Thatcher's speeches, as leader of the Conservative Party, reflected and reinforced this change of direction. She declared in 1976 that 'The mixed economy has become a nonsense phrase', which had been used to justify government's extensive intervention and which was responsible for the country's economic decline (Cooke 1989: 41). The Conservative Party manifesto in 1979 blamed it all on Labour because 'by enlarging the role of the state and diminishing the role of the individual, (Labour) have crippled the enterprise and effort on which a prosperous country with improving social services depends' (Conservative Party 1979: 6). It conveniently forgot the 30-year-long bipartisan approach to the welfare state and ignored the fact that the Labour Party, too, was beginning hesitantly to distance itself from the post-war conception of the universalist welfare state.

We shall be discussing Thatcherite ideas and policies in the 1980s in some detail in the next chapter. Here we merely sketch the Thatcherite approach to squaring the welfare circle. Basically, the new approach was based on three strategies: first, reduce the volume of public expenditure and expand the size of the national income; second, make the services fit into annually determined budgets; and third, privatise as many parts of welfare as was politically possible. Instead of accepting the size of the circle of services and then raising the resources to square the circle as previous governments had attempted to do, the Thatcher approach was to reverse the process. It attempted to determine the size of the square of resources and then match the circle of services to it. It had implications for many other aspects of life – poverty, inequality, taxation, trade union power, professionalisation, private provision, and so on – which we will discuss in the next chapter. That was the strategy, though it never worked all that well because of the electoral consequences of such a policy, the strong buoyancy of service demand – some of it created by government economic policies – the reduction of direct taxation rates, and the failure of the economy to rise to the occasion despite all Thatcherite proddings.

The Callaghan approach of the late 1970s had been at odds with that of most of the labour movement, who wished to carry on as before. In fact, the left of the labour movement argued for a more fundamental shift of government policies to transform the capitalist system. After three electoral defeats however, the Labour Party came to terms with the Callaghan philosophy. By the late 1980s, it came to accept that the growth in the economy was a major factor in determining the volume of public ex- penditure. Governments could no longer hope to finance expanding public service demand through rises in either public borrowing or direct taxation because, if for no other reason, the public had shown that it would not support such an approach. It thus came to accept 'realistic' limits to the expansion of social services and it also lowered its direct taxation rates, though not to the low level of Conservative governments. Naturally enough, it claimed that it could manage the economy better and thus produce the resources that are necessary to fulfil its ambitious social agenda based primarily on state provision. Its support for the universalist welfare state remained strong enough but its fiscal and economic policy proposals did not seem to be able to square the welfare circle completely.

The demise of Margaret Thatcher and the election of John Major as Prime Minister provided the last ingredient to this growing consensus. Major's forthright support of the public services and his 'citizen's charter' which sought to raise the quality of the services, to increase consumer choice, and to improve efficiency, seemed to move the Conservative Party away from the Thatcherite anti-welfare stance and to bring it closer to Labour on welfare issues. Both major parties now supported a form of welfare that was neither Thatcherite nor universalist. Some referred to it as the new 'social market consensus' (Haywood 1992: 74). We prefer to call it the 'affordable welfare state' to avoid the confusion which the term 'social market' generates.

In brief, the recession of the 1970s proved a watershed in the debates on squaring the welfare circle. On one hand, it marked the end of the post-war consensus on the universalist welfare state and, on the other, it ushered in a new paradigm – the affordable welfare state. The new paradigm was different from the old in at least five main ways. First, the volume of public expenditure must be closely determined by current rates of economic growth, as resources rather than needs are the overriding determinant of public expenditure. Second, direct taxation rates were to be as low as possible – although this was to be interpreted differently by the two main political parties. Third, the affordable welfare state implied a greater acceptance of private and voluntary provision both as supplements and as substitutes of state provision. In the social policy literature this came to be known as 'the mixed economy of welfare'. Fourth, public services should be managed in ways that they provide maximum value for money. Managerialism in public services was given a much higher profile than before. Fifth, the consumers of the services should have maximum feasible participation and choice. The power of the bureaucrats and of the professionals should be curbed as far as possible. These five strands of the new paradigm evolved gradually during the 1980s and they have now been accepted, to a greater or lesser extent, by the main political parties of the country. This does not signify total political consensus because agreement in principle does not necessarily mean agreement in the interpretation or implementation of these principles. Party political consensus and dissensus are as important now as they were under the previous welfare state paradigm. Party political agreement on the broad sweep of economic and social policy can never mean agreement on the specifics of policy – and the latter can often be of more significance than the former to the distributional effects of public policy.

As mentioned at the beginning of this chapter, the dilemmas of how to square the welfare circle are not unique to this country. They are common to all advanced industrial societies even though the solutions arrived at vary from one country to another. The social and economic changes that the British society went through during the 1950s and 1960s were pretty similar in all advanced industrial societies. Similarly, the recession of the late 1970s affected them all in varying ways and degrees. Thus the post-war consensus on the welfare state was under severe strain in all advanced industrial societies in the late 1970s, and the reason for this, as Mishra points out, 'were primarily "material" rather than ideational' (Mishra 1990: 1). National responses to this depended partly on the balance of political forces within countries. In other words, economic and political factors blended together to produce somewhat different responses in different countries. Some writers stress the similarity of responses, whilst others emphasise the differences. Padgett and Paterson point out that the new economic climate of the 1970s produced rather similar responses in Northern European countries. Economic discipline and restraint became the dominant government themes – and these did not fit well with the ideology of the left. They were themes where 'bourgeois parties held all the aces' (Padgett and Paterson 1991: 49). Mishra, on the other hand, outlines two types of such responses to the recession of the 1970s: neo-conservative responses on the right as in the USA, Canada, the UK, etc., and social corporatist approaches as in Sweden, Austria, Australia, etc. These two responses emerged in the 1980s as alternative approaches to, or at least as distinct departures from, the Keynesian welfare state (Mishra 1990: 76). Esping-Anderson extends the classification of welfare states during the 1980s to three ideal types, even though none of them is a 'pure case'. Each contains elements of the others (Esping-Anderson 1990: 28). They are, first, the social democratic regimes – the Scandinavian countries committed to universalist social services and full employment; second, the corporatist regimes of Austria, Germany, Italy and France stressing the provision of social rights to all groups without, however, seriously undermining their class structure; and third, the liberal welfare states of the USA, Canada, Australia and the UK in which 'means-tested assistance, modest universal transfers, or modest social-insurance plans predominate' (Esping-Anderson 1990: 26). The usefulness of the welfare state classifications for this discussion is that they show that different welfare state 'clusters' represent different attempts at squaring the welfare circle by reconciling the four main preoccupations of governments in advanced industrial societies outlined at the beginning of this chapter.

The first of these was the satisfaction of public demand for high quality social services. This public demand is influenced by a variety of factors, some of which are beyond the government's control. Demographic trends in relation to the retired population, social trends leading to the creation of one-parent families, marriage and remarriage rates, birth rates, improvements in living standards, and so on, all have policy implications and, on the whole, they create higher levels of service demand. Other factors leading to increased public expenditure are of the government's own making, directly or indirectly. Thatcherite policies for managing the economy during the 1980s inevitably led to sharp rises in unemployment which in turn had strong implications for government expenditures. Similarly concessions designed to improve a government's electoral chances are commonplace in all countries and for all parties. In brief, there is a structural web of interrelated social economic and political factors that individually and jointly make for higher rates of public expenditure which we discuss in Chapter 3.

Raising the necessary resources to meet this rising demand depends primarily on the rates of economic growth and on taxation. It is true that, for a while, governments can borrow or they can sell some of their assets to raise money or they can increase 'efficiency' in the public services, but these are temporary measures. In the long run, raising the necessary resources to square the circle of service demand has to rely on economic growth and taxation. This has now been accepted by all political parties in Britain and other industrial countries. Governments which maintain that many forms of public expenditure encourage economic growth will be prepared to argue the necessity of high taxation rates. On the other hand, governments which believe that high taxation rates inhibit economic growth are forced to rely even more on rates of economic growth only. Irrespective of the effects of taxation rates on economic growth, governments have also to take account of public opinion if they are to sustain their electoral chances. This is complicated by the fact that the public is more willing to pay indirect than direct taxes. It is for this reason that governments have tended to hold steady or reduce direct taxation rates but to increase indirect taxes during the past decade. Again, there are limits to which this can be done because of the effects of high indirect taxes on inflation and hence on economic growth. Governments which genuinely believe in a universalist welfare state have, therefore, a public education task on their hands: how to convince the various electoral groupings that better services may well mean high taxation rates as well. Governments which believe in a minimal welfare state have an equally difficult political task. The welfare state has deep roots in this country, nourished not simply by ideology but by self-interest as well. It has conferred benefits on all groups in varying ways and degrees and, in several respects, it has proved indispensable to economic growth. All this highlights the severe political and economic constraints of squaring the welfare circle. In a democracy, party political ideology has to be trimmed and compromised in the rough-and-tumble of everyday politics and in the pursuit of political power. Chapter 2 will show that even the most ideological of governments had to submit to this iron law of political life in a parliamentary democracy.

This chapter has traced debates on squaring the welfare circle in Britain from the 1940s to the 1990s. It has shown that the political consensus underpinning the Keynesian–Beveridgean universal welfare state was undermined by material factors which led to the emergence of a new paradigm – the affordable welfare state – that now commands considerable bipartisan support. Like all other paradigms, the affordable welfare state delineates and legitimises the main courses of action open to political parties contesting for government but it is also vague and flexible enough to make party political dissensus also inevitable. Thus, though the two main political parties subscribe to similar, though not identical, approaches for squaring the welfare circle, they are also divided on a host of issues which are not mere matters of detail but of real substance, for they have different implications for different groups in society as the discussion in the following chapters will show. The 1992 election demonstrated both how predominant the idea of the affordable welfare state had become and how important the differences that remained between the parties could be. Labour's modest proposals for increased taxation to support welfare became perhaps the greatest issue of the campaign, although, as we shall see, it remained unclear how costly – if indeed at all – these proposals were in electoral terms.

The welfare conundrum of the twenty-first century is now pretty clear. Can generous social provision be combined with low taxation at times of low or even modest rates of economic growth, or is the new affordable welfare state likely to become increasingly unaffordable?

Chapter 2

The Thatcherite attempt to square the circle

Vic George and Stewart Miller

The debate we have described was coming to a head in the late 1970s, as the Callaghan government struggled to square the circle in the wake of the 1976 crisis and in the context of the monetarism imposed by the International Monetary Fund at that time. But the election that brought the Thatcher administration into existence in 1979 was fought largely on the ground of industrial relations, particularly in the public sector, and 'Thatcherism' was a term scarcely dreamt of. Nevertheless, it quickly became clear that the intention of the new government was to pursue policies that on the one hand would maximise the rate of economic growth, and on the other would reduce the supply of and demand for freely provided social services. Thus the government would achieve the resolution that had eluded all previous post-war governments – it would square the welfare circle, breaking the cycle of increasing provision and increasing demand that Mrs Thatcher and her colleagues saw as an intolerable drain on economic resources. In this chapter we examine the record of the Thatcher governments in seeking this goal, considering both the means adopted and the degree of success enjoyed. We begin with the economic context of social policy, asking whether there was or was not an 'economic miracle'; then we narrow the discussion down to the specific central issue of public expenditure, looking at the techniques used for controlling this and the extent to which the strategy proved successful; and finally we consider the impact of all these factors on service performance and standards, on poverty and inequality, and on popular opinion and values.

THE ECONOMIC RECORD: MIRACLE OR MIRAGE?

In order to assess the Thatcherite record on the economy, we will examine the performance of five main indicators: labour productivity, the balance of payments, inflation, unemployment and, to begin with, gross domestic product (GDP). In terms of GDP growth, the 1980s were disappointing compared with previous post-war decades. The average annual rate of growth in the 1960s and 1970s was 3.1 per cent and 2.4 per cent respectively, whereas in the 1980s it was 1.9 per cent according to Coutts and Godley and 2.1 per cent according to the OECD (Coutts and Godley 1989: 138; OECD 1989: 58). Table 2.1 compares British average annual growth with that of other members of the 'Group of Seven' leading industrial countries in the 1970s and 1980s. It shows that British performance was worse than all the others in the 1970s and still worse than most in the 1980s, although there was some relative improvement.

Equally important for future economic prosperity is labour productivity, since this influences heavily the competitiveness of the country in the international market. As Table 2.2 shows, British productivity grew faster in the 1980s than in the years 1973–9, and came a little closer to the Group of Seven average. Within this, there was real improvement in the 1980s in the manufacturing sector, where growth reached 4.2 per cent, the highest figure in the Group of Seven. But these improvements took place alongside radical shrinkage in the size of the manufacturing sector and a dramatic rise in unemployment.

Despite the substantial revenues from North Sea oil, the trade balance of the country remained a problem. In 1986, after six years of surpluses averaging £3 billion a year, the trade balance turned into a mild deficit, which then rose sharply to reach a record high of £19.6 billion in 1989. As a proportion of GDP, the British balance of payments deficit in the late 1980s was higher

Table 2.1 Average annual percentage growth in GDP

	UK	USA	Japan	Germany	France	Italy	Canada
1970s	2.4	2.8	5.4	3.1	3.7	3.9	4.7
1980s	2.3	2.7	4.2	1.9	2.1	2.5	3.2

Source: Adapted from OECD 1990a: 181

Table 2.2 Annual percentage growth in output per person in employment

	Whole economy			Manufacturing		
	1960–73	1973–9	1979–88	1960–73	1973–9	1979–88
UK	2.6	1.1	1.9	3.6	0.7	4.2
USA	1.9	0.0	0.8	3.8	1.8	3.3
Japan	8.2	2.9	3.0	8.9	3.4	2.4
Germany	4.2	2.9	1.6	4.5	2.5	1.4
France	4.7	2.5	1.9	4.9	2.6	2.1
Italy	5.7	1.8	1.6	5.9	2.5	2.9
Canada	2.4	1.3	1.1	3.5	1.0	2.2
Average[1]	4.2	1.5	1.6	4.9	2.4	3.0

Source: OECD 1989: 58
Note: [1] 1987 weights

than that of most industrial countries, and on a par with the constantly high level of the USA (Coutts and Godley 1989: 140).

Turning to the Thatcher government's highest priority, the control of inflation, the record is impressive only when compared to the notorious 1970s. Bazen and Thirlwall have provided evidence of a secular trend of rising inflation for most of the post-war period, regardless of the political nature of the government. Thus between 1951 and 1964, when the Conservatives were in power, inflation averaged 3.5 per cent per annum; during the Labour period of 1964–70, 5.2 per cent; and for the Conservative period of 1970–4, 11.2 per cent. In 1974–9, with Labour in office again, it shot up to 21.2 per cent; and the figure of 8.4 per cent for 1979–89 is certainly an improvement on that. But again, as Table 2.3 shows, comparison with the other major industrial countries makes this improvement look relatively modest (Bazen and Thirlwall 1989).

The 1980s witnessed unprecedented post-war rates of unemployment. In fact, the government used unemployment as an

Table 2.3 Percentage rise in consumer prices

	UK	USA	Japan	Germany	France	Italy	Canada
1968–77	12.1	6.4	9.7	4.9	8.3	10.9	6.7
1977–89	8.0	6.2	2.8	3.0	7.9	11.9	7.0

Source: OECD 1990a: 130

Table 2.4 Standardised unemployment rates (per cent)

	UK	USA	Japan	Germany	France	Italy	Canada
1970–9	4.3	6.1	1.7	2.3	3.8	6.2	6.6
1980–9	10.0	7.2	2.5	6.0	9.0	9.5	9.3

Source: OECD 1990a: 130

instrument for curbing trade union power and controlling inflation. Britain topped the Group of Seven league for unemployment in the 1980s (see Table 2.4), and continued to experience 'stagflation' – the combination of inflation with low growth and high unemployment.

Overall, the 1980s saw an improvement over the 1960s and 1970s in productivity growth; deterioration in GDP growth, the balance of payments and unemployment; and an improvement in inflation relative only to the 1970s. Britain continued to compare unfavourably with its major competitors in GDP growth, trade and unemployment. There was little evidence at the time to support the Chancellor of the Exchequer's 1988 claim of 'an economic miracle' comparable to those of West Germany and Japan; and the subsequent performance of the economy positively mocked such ideas. It is quite evident that the government could not possibly square the welfare circle through economic growth and could only hope to do so through reductions in the need and demand for public services.

PUBLIC EXPENDITURE

Cutting public expenditure was seen as a means of improving economic performance, as well as in itself a goal of a government dedicated to restricting the role of the state. Public services were perceived to be in competition with private investment both for revenue (through taxation) and for capital (through borrowing); this competition enhanced demand for money and so inflation. Moreover, public services competed with private industry for labour, and forced up labour costs. Finally, an excess of free or heavily subsidised services undermined the market forces which were thought to be the motive force of productive activity. The growth of spending on social provision was seen as having got out of hand .

The monetarist attitude was set out in the 1979 White Paper,

The Government's Expenditure Plans, 1980–81, which declared that
'Public expenditure is at the heart of Britain's present economic
difficulties' (HM Treasury 1979: 1). 'Over the years,' the White
Paper continued, 'public spending has been increased on assumptions about economic growth which have not been achieved. The
inevitable result has been a growing burden of taxes and
borrowing' (1979: 2). In other words, governments had failed to
square the circle. Immediate objectives were to reduce inflation,
to restore incentives by holding down and if possible reducing
taxes, and to 'stabilise' public spending.

> Higher output can only come from lower taxes, lower interest
> rates and less Government borrowing, and better use of
> investment. To plan more public services before the required
> output is available to support it would ensure that, in the event,
> that growth of output does not take place. Higher public
> expenditure cannot any longer be allowed to precede, and thus
> prevent, growth in the private sector.
>
> (HM Treasury 1979: 2)

These were to be the considerations dominating the Thatcher
government's approach to public expenditure and to social policy
for the next eleven years. They were not new; both Conservative
and Labour governments had said similar things at various times.
But now the determination to act upon these principles was
shored up by the theoretical underpinning of monetarism and the
psychological prop of a singularly determined Prime Minister.

Methods and techniques of containment

The attempt to control and restrain public expenditure took a
variety of forms and used a variety of methods. The new
assumption was that public services would gobble up anything you
let them have, so it was necessary to keep their allocations firmly
in check and, as far as possible, leave it to service managers to
make the difficult decisions that followed. Some restraint methods
stem directly from that strategy; others draw on other strands of
the overall approach of Thatcherism. The particular methods we
draw attention to here are: cash management, devolved budgeting, revenue structuring, privatisation, marketisation, charging,
targeting and incentives. Of course, several of these overlap.

The government's determination to make finance determine

provision led to technical changes in public expenditure planning, intended to set up a new and restrictive framework for all future spending decisions. This was not done from scratch. In particular, planning in terms of the volume of services had already been modified across much of the range by the introduction of cash limits – specific annual financial ceilings through which spending in a particular area could not go, regardless of increases in costs within the year. When the Thatcher government took over, cash limits for particular years existed alongside a system of year-on-year planning which continued to express monies 'in real terms', adjusting for inflation in the past and assuming similar adjustments in the future. This was not to the taste of a government which saw inflation as its greatest problem. The failure of its early attempts to restrict public spending growth convinced the Conservative government – and its natural ally, the Treasury – that closer control was necessary (Thain and Wright 1990: 160). From 1981, therefore, the government did its expenditure planning in cash terms – actual numbers of pounds to be made available – making such allowances about future inflation as it deemed appropriate but declining to guarantee the adjustment of promised monies to cover rises in costs. Moreover, with cash planning the new norm, the system of cash limits was progressively extended into realms, such as parts of the health service, where such limits had previously been thought inappropriate on grounds of acute need. As we shall see, by the end of the decade cash limits had even made an appearance in the area of social security.

Other techniques aimed at structuring future spending decisions sprang logically from the cash planning/cash limits system. With the volume of services now determined by strictly limited finance, it seemed to make more sense to attempt less detailed control of service provision on the ground, and better to devolve responsibility along with the money and leave it to the local managers to square their own, smaller circles. This strategy was followed in the worlds of education and health care, culminating in the 'devolved budgeting' provisions in the Acts of (respectively) 1988 and 1989. Local schools and hospitals gained increased control of their own expenditure, and degrees of freedom to seek finance outside the public sphere, at the cost of losing much contingent protection by their supervising authorities.

A further, related technique was that of structuring the process of revenue-raising in such a way as to build in a bias against growth. The Community Charge (or 'poll tax') was the most notorious example of this. It was the centre-piece of the reform of local government finance and a replacement for the local property tax on housing, the domestic 'rates'. The new, personal tax was designed to make as conspicuous as possible to local voters the consequences of electing high-spending administrations, and to ensure that no one should be in the position of enjoying services for which they were not helping to pay. It was to be an automatic aid to squaring the circle in local services. But the new system failed to act as automatically as its designers had hoped. Voters blamed central government for imposing the tax on them, rather than local leaderships for levying it; central government could not bring itself to wait for the 'poll tax effect' to work, but activated measures of control on local charge levels which destroyed at once the automation and the government's own concept of local accountability; and the 'simple' poll tax, widely perceived as unfair and oppressive, proved impossibly difficult to collect. After Mrs Thatcher's fall the government quickly moved to replace it, returning to a property-based levy in the new Council Tax.

It would have been surprising if privatisation had not been an important element in the strategy to contain public expenditure. By 'privatisation', we mean both the withdrawal of the state from areas of provision through selling off public assets or winding up public organisations, and the transfer of actual service provision from the public to the private sector, even where it continues to be publicly financed. The latter overlaps with another, vitally important strategy: the introduction of markets within the public sector and in the interfaces between the public and the private sectors.

Housing was an area where the government pursued more than one strategy of privatisation: they sold public housing both to its tenants and to private landlords. One of the few distinctly 'Thatcherite' policies flagged in the 1979 Conservative manifesto, granting council tenants the right to buy their own houses at dis-counted prices (Conservative Party 1979: 23–4), proved enormously popular. The next stage in the assault on the public housing sector, the attempted wholesale transfer of local authority blocks or estates to 'the independent sector', was less spectacularly successful.

Another privatisation tactic involved social security, and the redefinition of basic assumptions about the role of the state in pension provision. The Thatcher government's 1985 Green Paper took the line that if more pensioners were to be removed from means testing, what was required was not more universal state benefits but more alternatives to state benefits. Opposition to the complete abandonment of the State Earnings Related Pension Scheme (SERPS) led to a compromise by which it was made less attractive and the transfer to private arrangements subsidised heavily. Younger people in stable jobs are now better off contracting with private pension schemes than staying in SERPS, although the collapse of Robert Maxwell's chain of companies and associated pension funds showed how vulnerable such forms of provision can be – when they are not closely regulated by government.

Before the substantial privatisation of mainstream social services was thought to be possible, the government contented itself with the 'contracting out' of ancillary services such as cleaning and catering in state hospitals, schools and other institutions. Sometimes this took the form of contracting with private firms, to provide services to the service authority, as when competitive tendering was used for cleaning. Sometimes services such as catering or running shops within institutions were taken over by private firms, which then entered into market relations with the user public. The gains brought about by such developments remain matters of dispute, not only among those concerned with quality of service – see our discussion of this in this and the final chapter – but among such groups as the public sector trade unions whose members' jobs were lost or devalued in the process.

Le Grand (1982) considers the most important departure from the traditional pattern of social policy provision to be the construction of market relations within public provision, largely by pricing transfers of resource within the service. It was education that first felt the impact of this new approach, with a series of detailed changes in school and college funding during the 1980s, culminating in the Education Reform Act of 1988 and the White Papers of 1991 on post-16 education and training. The principle was, on the whole, that schools and colleges be funded according to their success in attracting students, with far fewer guarantees of continuity of finance. But the best-known example of marketisation in the canon of late Thatcherite reforms was the introduction into the National Health Service of an 'internal market' system, with budget holders and service providers sufficiently divorced for a set of market relations to exist between them, bringing incentives to efficiency through competition, both among themselves and with potential rivals from outside (Department of Health 1989). Another market whose creation was promised in the same legislation of 1990 which enacted the NHS reform was that in community care, although that was one whose realisation was delayed. All of these examples are discussed in later chapters.

All these changes took place alongside other, more orthodox conservative measures to increase the selectivity of social services. Charging users for services, for instance, is an obvious strategy for a government with faith in the workings of the market. It is seen not only as a source of revenue but as a rationing device, deterring frivolous or spurious use of scarce resources. Examples of the charging strategy are rife in primary health care. Drug prescription charges were enormously increased, and charges introduced, to the accompaniment of much criticism, for dental and optical checks in addition to treatments. The concern caused by this move has been reinforced by subsequent evidence of a decline in use of such checks.

We have already referred to pension reform; this was part of a broader social security strategy to systematise what was seen as the inevitably large means-tested element of social security. The selectivity of Housing Benefit was enhanced, and the 'special needs' element of social security was given over to the new Social Fund. That this represented an entirely different approach from past policy was emphasised, not only by its emphasis on loans rather than grants, but also by its having a limited budget – an innovation for social security.

The 1986 Social Security Act, and its justification in the preceding Green and White Papers, was also characterised by a concern to 'target' benefits to those thought to be in greatest need. Negatively, some relatively better-off groups of benefit recipients, and some seen as less deserving (such as young people thought to be able to rely on their families), were excluded from eligibility; positively, the new pattern of benefits was designed to enhance the support of families with children – although, in practice, these two sides of the policy frequently clashed.

Related to targeting, but not always entirely compatible with it, was the attempt to protect and promote incentives which would reduce dependence on benefits and other public services. This was another of the main aims of the 1986 Social Security Act: to ensure that the pattern of social security provision did not unduly discourage people from actively entering and staying in the labour force. The relative attractiveness of combining wages with Family Credit over remaining on Income Support was intended to act as a better incentive than the former arrangements.

Thus the expenditure-controlling strategy of the Thatcher government was characterised by a tremendous variety of measures, intended to undermine the received wisdom and assumptions of the post-war welfare state concerning expenditure growth, provision and entitlement; and radically to alter the practice and performance of the public social services.

Rise and fall

What, then, happened to public expenditure during the Thatcher years? Was the burden which it was seen to present lessened, or its distribution substantially changed? We shall begin with the story told by the expenditure White Paper of 1990 (Mrs Thatcher's last year as Prime Minister) from which Table 2.5 is taken.

In view of the resolve of the government to check the growth of public expenditure it is interesting to note that that growth did not cease over this period. Between 1978–9 and 1989–90, public expenditure on services, taking inflation into account, rose by 16.7 per cent; 1.4 per cent per year on average. Privatisation proceeds, for arcane reasons, appear in government accounts as negative expenditure rather than as income. These help to reduce the rise in overall expenditure to 13.4 per cent over the period; but they never amounted to more than £7.5bn in any one year.

Table 2.5 General government expenditure in real terms (£bn) (base 1989–90)

	1978–9	1983–4	1989–90
General government expenditure	175.4	193.7	198.9
Expenditure on services	152.7	169.2	178.2
of which:			
Social security	39.6	50.6	52.9
Housing	10.7	6.2	4.8
Health and personal social services	21.6	25.2	29.5
Education and science	22.2	22.6	25.1

Source: HM Treasury 1989

Of course, not all the public services rose and fell together. Concentrating on social provision, we can see clear contrasts in the fortunes of different parts of the welfare state. By far the largest single area of public expenditure is social security, representing some 30 per cent of all public service spending. Social security rose by a third during the ten years we are considering. Most of that increase took place during the years of growing unemployment up to 1983, reflecting the fact that social security is paid out largely in response to claims of right triggered by specific contingencies, and cannot be budgeted downwards as readily as other services. Rights can, of course, be reduced, and there was a late downturn reflecting the cuts in entitlement brought about by the 1986 Social Security Act, to which we have referred. But the growth in unemployment, the elderly population and lone-parent families threaten to keep social security spending relatively high.

Contrast this with the fate of housing. Already singled out for cut-backs by the previous government, housing expenditure was slashed under Thatcher, falling by 1989–90 to less than half of its 1978–9 level. Under both the 1980 and 1988 Acts some housing expenditure was transferred to social security, but this by no means explains the extraordinary scale of reduction achieved in this area. General subsidies to public house building effectively ceased, and the relative and absolute size of the public housing sector itself was cut substantially through council house sales and the government's refusal to sanction public building.

Health and personal social service spending went up by 36.6 per cent and education and science by 13 per cent. Although these services are in some degree budgetable, they are also subject to demographic influences which, on the one hand, boosted the elderly proportion of the population that provides the National Health Service and local social services with much of their business and, on the other hand, shrunk the proportion of the young, for whom education is largely demanded. Much of spending in all of these services is on people as providers, so the industrial and political difficulties of cutting back are far greater than in housing.

Table 2.6 helps us to assess the record of the Thatcher government in comparison with its two predecessors. These were the Heath Conservative administration, in office from 1970 to 1974, and the Labour government of 1974 to 1979, led by Harold Wilson and then by James Callaghan. The figures are of the

Table 2.6 Total outlays of government as percentage of GDP

	1970	1975	1980	1989
UK	38.8	46.6	44.9	41.2
USA	31.6	34.6	33.7	36.1
Japan	19.4	27.3	32.6	31.5
Germany	38.6	48.9	48.3	45.5
France	38.5	43.4	46.1	49.4
Italy	34.2	43.2	41.7	51.5
Canada	34.8	40.1	40.5	44.6
Total	32.3	37.7	38.4	38.7

Source: OECD 1992: Table R15.

OECD's concept of 'total outlays of government', a slightly broader concept than either 'expenditure on services' or 'general government expenditure', including as it does gross capital formation. But the relativities remain valid and interesting.

While we have seen that UK public expenditure grew in money terms during the Thatcher era, it is clear that it did decline slightly as a proportion of the GDP. (The difference is the result of growth in the economy amounting to 19 per cent: OECD 1990a.) This was a reversal of the overall trend of the 1970s, although there were more fluctuations than are shown in Table 2.6: 1975 and 1984 (47.5 per cent) were both peak years. The relative spending growth of the 1970s is by no means untypical of Western industrial countries – broadly, the membership of the OECD – of major industrial economies, or of the countries of the European Community. But the marginal reversal of that trend in the overall figure for the 1980s is more unusual, although many other countries had also passed their peak of proportionate spending by 1987.

The Thatcher government used the declining ratio of its outlays to the GDP partly to reduce direct taxation (although it actually increased indirect taxation substantially) and partly to reduce its borrowing requirement. By 1988, the annual budget was no longer running the deficit characteristic of Western states in the Keynesian era, and particularly in the difficult period of the late 1970s and the early 1980s, and was showing a surplus in its general financial balance of over 1 per cent of the GDP. (Of the six major OECD countries with which the UK is compared above, only Japan in 1987 and 1988 and the United States in 1979 had experienced a surplus since the distant days of 1975 (OECD 1990a: 194).) However, the economic circumstances of the late 1980s and early 1990s undermined this budgetary achievement, and the successors of the Thatcher government were, by 1992, learning to live with budget deficits at least pro tem, and explaining that they could be tolerated during a recession.

Thus the government may be said to have met, to some extent, its objective of lowering the demands both of direct taxation and of public borrowing on the economy; but not to have wrought an irreversible change, at least on the latter count. Indeed, if one takes account of indirect taxation, the Thatcher government could not claim to have reduced the overall burden of taxation at all:

> In 1979 the Conservative government collected 35% of the national output in taxes. By 1990, despite the government's much-trumpeted cuts in rates of income tax, the overall tax burden had actually gone up, to 38%.
>
> (*The Economist*, 18 May 1991: 19)

We shall return to this point later: it emphasises the difficulty of squaring the welfare circle, even for a government without a strong ideological welfare commitment – in this case, indeed, quite the reverse.

THE IMPACT OF THE THATCHERITE ATTEMPT TO SQUARE THE CIRCLE

The strategies we have described, specific and general, were intended to amount to a transformation of the public services and the culture that was thought to have sustained inefficiency and indiscrimination in them. Here we attempt to gauge their impact on social services, on inequality and on public opinion and culture. First, we review some aspects of the social service performance of the 1980s and compare that performance with that of the previous decade across a range of inputs and immediate outputs.

The performance of the social services

We have already observed that housing was the area where the severest expenditure cuts were made in the 1980s. Here, the most publicised change has been the shift from public renting to home ownership resulting directly from government policies. But more important is the growth of the housing stock required to cater for increased housing need stemming from the rising number of households, particularly in areas of high population growth. Judged by this criterion, the record of the 1980s is near dismal. Between 1971 and 1980, on average, the annual net addition to the housing stock was 302,000. For the nine years from 1981 to 1989 the figure was 196,000: a marked slowing down of growth at a time when the number of households increased faster due to such phenomena as rising divorce and separation rates, rising numbers of students and other young people living away from home, and so on. It is a record that will continue to cause severe housing difficulties in the future.

Notwithstanding important party political differences, housing policy has always had one fundamental objective: to ensure that 'all families should be able to obtain a decent home at a price within their means' (DoE 1977: 1). Table 2.7 uses very basic criteria to evaluate housing policy in the 1980s. It shows that in terms of such amenities as baths, toilets and heating, the 1980s witnessed a rate of improvement which was slower than that of the 1970s. In terms of the harshest of physical standards, the 1980s were as unsuccessful as the 1970s in reducing the number of dwellings that were either unfit or in serious disrepair. What characterised the 1980s, however, was the sharp rise in home-

Table 2.7 Basic amenities, overcrowding and homelessness in Great Britain

	1971	1981	1988
Percentage with sole use of bath or shower	88	96	98
Percentage with central heating	35	59	76
Percentage below bedroom standard	9	5	3
Thousands of unfit dwellings	1,250	1,200	1,100
Thousands of dwellings in serious disrepair	1,100	1,200	1,250
Thousands of households rehoused as homeless by local authorities	–	86	175
Thousands of houses repossessed by mortgage lenders because of arrears	–	5	44[1]
Thousands of families in mortgage arrears of 6–12 months	–	25	123[1]

Sources: for 1–6: CSO 1991: 139, Table 8.10, and 140, Table 8.13. For 7 and 8: Smithers 1991
Note: [1] Refers to 1990

lessness and housing indebtedness. The figures on homelessness grossly underestimate the seriousness of the problem because they exclude those sleeping rough, those sharing accommodation against their wishes and, above all, most of the single homeless estimated at 124,000 in 1989 (Greve 1990: 90). In policy terms, the rise in homelessness suggests that reliance on the market not only cannot satisfy the housing needs of the most vulnerable groups in society but indeed increases the volume of that need.

We have already seen that the sharp rise in social security expenditure was accompanied by an almost equal rise in the numbers of people with incomes below the Income Support level. The explanation for this seeming paradox is that the increase in expenditure was due solely to the rise in the number of people receiving benefits and not to any improvement in the level of benefits. Indeed, the main social security benefits declined in value relative to the gross earnings of all adult male workers in full-time employment. Unemployment Benefit and Supplementary Benefit/Income Support continued in the 1980s the relative decline of the 1970s: the standard rate of Supplementary Benefit, 26.6 per cent of average male earnings in 1971, was 25.3 per cent in 1981 and 19.5 per cent (for the equivalent benefit) in 1990 (DSS 1990a: 281–92). Retirement pensions, which had improved relatively in the 1970s, shared in the decline of the 1980s: the basic pension for a couple went down from 31.7 per cent of average male earnings in 1981 to 25.4 per cent in 1990 (1990a: 281–92). These figures take no account of additions for housing costs, and the changes introduced in the 1980s un- questionably mean that the relative value of benefits including housing additions effectively declined much more. Even relative to prices, benefits also declined in value during the 1980s. At April 1990 prices, the basic retirement pension for a single person was worth £47.60 in 1981 and £46.90 in 1990. On the other hand, a small proportion of beneficiaries did very well during the 1980s as a result of taxation policy changes and improved occupational pensions. The 'two nations in old age' that Titmuss referred to in 1955 grew even further apart during the 1980s (Titmuss 1955: 152–66).

In education, there are a number of key statistics that begin to indicate trends in standards. Table 2.8 shows continued improve-ment in pupil:teacher ratios and size of classes. But whereas the progress of the 1970s was achieved mainly through the employ-ment of more teachers, that of the 1980s came about through

Table 2.8 Education service standards in the UK

	1970–1	1980–1	1988–9
Pupil:teacher ratio, primary schools	27.1	22.3	21.9
Pupil:teacher ratio, secondary schools	17.8	16.4	15.9
Percentage of classes with 31 or more pupils, primary	34	22	17
Percentage of classes with 31 or more pupils, secondary	12	8	4
Average size of class, primary	28	26	26
Average size of class, secondary	22	22	21
Percentage of teachers with graduate status, primary	7	17	27
Percentage of teachers with graduate status, secondary	39	54	60
£ expenditure per primary pupil at 1988–9 prices	–	870	1,102
£ expenditure per secondary pupil at 1988–9 prices	–	1,217	1,692
Capital spending on schools, £bn at 1988–9 prices	–	1.2	0.9

Sources: for 1, 2, 7 and 8: DES 1989: Table A, p.iv and Table H, p.xi; for 11: Fielding 1990; for 3–6, 9 and 10: CSO 1991: 50, Table 3.9 and 62, Table 3.35

declining numbers of pupils. The total number of teachers in primary and secondary schools rose from 402,000 in 1970 to 503,000 in 1980, but declined to 459,000 in 1987 (DES 1989: xi). The quality of teachers in terms of graduate status continued to rise during the 1980s, though at a slower rate than in the previous decade. Nevertheless, shortages of qualified teachers in specific subjects such as science, mathematics and modern languages continued in the 1980s and were repeatedly referred to by HM Inspectorate of Schools. Education spending per capita of the population continued to rise, even if this was at a much slower rate in higher education than was warranted by the increase in the number of students. However, it was the budget on school building construction and maintenance that suffered severely in the 1980s, with detrimental effects. The 1990 Report of the Senior Chief Inspector of Schools expressed serious concern regarding secondary school buildings. The Inspectorate 'judged two-thirds of the schools inspected to have unsuitable accommodation and in just less than half of those the problems were serious and adversely affecting the quality of the work in one way or another'

Table 2.9 Outcome standards of education in the UK

	1970–1	1980–1	1988–9
Percentage of school-leavers with 2 or more A-level passes			
Boys	15	15	16
Girls	13	13	16
Full-time students in higher education (thousands)			
Male	254.2	277.7	308.7
Female	178.1	203.9	270.4

Source: CSO 1991: 50, Table 3.12, and 56, Table 3.19

(HM Senior Chief Inspector of Schools 1990: 3). Moreover, the Report referred to shortages of school equipment and 'shortcomings in the quantity of books available as well as in their appropriateness' (1990: 10).

Table 2.9 shows some education outcomes. There was a significant improvement in the achievement of girls in higher education in the 1980s, but overall the UK continues to lag behind most comparable European countries in terms of the qualifications of education-leavers. Evidence about the failures of the system, such as school-leavers who do not reach adequate standards of literacy or numeracy, is hard to come by in any consistent form that makes possible comparisons over time.

The 1980s witnessed a number of changes in the health services, as is clear from Table 2.10. The first was a lengthening of hospital waiting lists; about 25 per cent of those on these lists had been waiting for treatment for over twelve months in 1990. Nevertheless the number of people treated as in-patients increased. The second was the shortening of doctors' and dentists' patient lists, a continuation of previous trends. This, however, must be seen in the light of higher proportions of the very elderly and deteriorating provision in inner city areas, particularly London.

It is impossible to write about trends in social service standards without commenting briefly on the relevance of rising public aspirations and of social class inequalities. Rising standards in housing, education and health inevitably create demands. It is natural, for example, that an increasing proportion of parents, having experienced higher education, will demand more and better education for their children. In this respect relative dissatisfaction with social service provision is natural and

Table 2.10 Health service standards in the UK

	1971	1981	1988–9
Average number of hospital beds available daily (thousands)	526	450	373
Average number of hospital beds occupied daily (thousands)	436	366	304
Patients treated per bed available	12.3	16.0	21.8
Hospital in-patient waiting lists (thousands)	700.8[1]	736.6	841.6[2]
Doctors in practice (thousands)	24.0	27.5	31.5
Patients per doctor (thousands)	2.39	2.15	1.91
Percentage of doctors' lists above 2,500 in England	47.0	28.0	11.4
Percentage of doctors' lists above 3,000 in England	19.0	6.3	2.3
Number of dentists in practice (thousands)	12.5	15.2	18.4
Patients per dentist (thousands)	4.5	3.7	2.1

Source: CSO 1991: 128, Tables 7.31 and 7.32, and 129, Table 7.33. For doctors' lists: DoH 1973, 1982, 1990
Notes: [1] Refers to 1976; [2] refers to 1990

constructive. As Crosland remarked twenty years ago, 'a modern welfare state, by continuously raising its standards, ensures that it always falls short of its own expectations' (Crosland 1974: 23). Some of the shortfalls of social service provision can be so explained – but there are others, particularly in housing, where the deterioration in meeting needs was absolute and of a different order.

The improvement of standards should not be confused with reductions of inequalities, of class, gender or race. It is well known that social class and ethnicity correlate with differences in housing standards. In 1988, after a period of growth in owner occupation, 89 per cent of the professional classes were home owners compared to 35 per cent of unskilled manual workers. The worst housing conditions are in the privately-rented sector where concentrations of the lowest socio-economic groups and certain ethnic groups are to be found. Thus, while only 1 per cent of white households were grossly overcrowded in 1988, the corresponding proportion among non-white households was 9 per cent (CSO 1991: 139). Similarly, the expansion of higher education in the 1980s did not result in a reduction of social class difference. Nor did the reduction in mortality rates among young children reduce the gap between the higher and the lower socio-economic groups,

Table 2.11 Social policy and social class inequalities in the UK

Social class (see note below for category)	I	II	III(a)	III(b)	IV	V
Per cent of university students admitted, 1980–1	22.3	47.8	10.4	14.0	4.4	1.0
Per cent of university students admitted, 1988–9	20.7	49.2	10.9	12.1	6.1	1.1
Perinatal mortality per 1,000 births, 1978–9	11.9	12.3	13.9	15.1	16.7	20.3
Perinatal mortality per 1,000 births, 1987–8	6.8	7.0	7.8	8.1	9.9	10.8
Infant mortality per 1,000 births, 1978–9	9.8	10.1	11.1	12.4	13.6	17.2
Infant mortality per 1,000 births, 1987–8	6.9	6.7	7.1	7.7	9.6	11.8

Sources: For university students, UCCA 1990: 5; for mortality rates, Oppenheim 1990: 58, Table 11
Note: I: Professional occupations. II: Intermediate occupations. III(a): Skilled occupations: non-manual. III(b): Skilled occupations: manual. IV: Partly skilled occupations. V: Unskilled occupations

as Table 2.11 shows. Clearly, reductions in class differentials require policy measures that explicitly and strongly favour the 'ower socio-economic groups – a strategy that runs counter both to dominant values and to dominant interests in society.

Inequality and poverty

The strong emphasis on monetary incentives as a stimulus to productivity in fiscal and economic policies had the expected result of increasing inequalities. So did the reduction in the relative level of social security benefits, aimed at strengthening work incentives. It came to be seen as axiomatic that the highly paid needed positive monetary incentives while those on benefits could best be motivated to greater effort through negative financial sanctions. Thus pay awards and changes in personal taxation rates and in benefit levels combined to widen the gap between those on high and those on low incomes. This conclusion stands whether one looks at earnings from work or income in general.

Take, for example, the dispersion of incomes from work for full-time male manual workers, for which we have data going back a long way. The range in 1886 went from 68.6 per cent of the median for the lowest decile to 143.1 per cent for the highest, and in 1979 from 68.3 per cent to 148.5 per cent, showing remarkable stability. Change was much more dramatic in the 1980s, leaving the lowest decile in 1990 earning 63.71 per cent of the median and the highest decile 159.1 per cent (LPU 1991: 11–13).

A very similar picture emerges if one looks specifically at the earnings of all low-paid full-time workers. The risk of low pay has always been higher among women, but the policies of the 1980s particularly affected the position of low-paid men: the proportion of men whose wages fell below the Council of Europe's decency threshold almost doubled, from 14.6 per cent to 28.1 per cent, while that of women fell slightly, but remained over 50 per cent (LPU 1991: 11–13).

In terms of income from all sources, the trend is again towards greater inequality (see Table 2.12). The incomes of all groups rose in the 1980s, but at a higher rate for the top than for the lower income groups. Indeed, the only group whose share of total income increased was that of the top 20 per cent of income earners. Moreover, these figures do not take account of the value of fringe benefits, which is much higher for this group than for others. Finally, the changes in taxation rates and the restrictions of social security benefits introduced in the 1980s are likely further to enhance these inequalities.

While income inequalities increased during the 1980s wealth inequalities did not, due primarily to the rise in home ownership and the sale of shares in the privatisation of such industries as gas, electricity, water and telephones. It is clear from Table 2.13 that the redistribution of wealth that took place during the decade was from the rich to the merely well-off. The top 10 per cent of wealth owners commanded 50 per cent of the country's marketable wealth in 1979 and 53 per cent in 1988. Indeed, the bottom half

Table 2.12 Distribution of pre-tax and post-tax income of UK households (per cent)

| Quintile group | Pre-tax income | | Post-tax income | |
	1979	1987	1979	1987
Bottom group	0.5	0.3	6.1	5.1
Second group	9	6	11	10
Third group	19	16	18	16
Fourth group	27	27	25	24
Top group	45	51	40	45
Total	100	100	100	100

Source: DE 1990

Table 2.13 Distribution of marketable wealth among adults in the UK (per cent)

Population group	1979	1986	1988 (est.)
Top 1%	20	18	17
Top 2%	26	24	25
Top 5%	37	36	38
Top 10%	50	50	53
Top 25%	72	73	75
Top 50%	92	90	94
Bottom 50%	8	10	6

Source: Board of Inland Revenue 1990: 103, Table 10.5

of the population lost out and their share, only 8 per cent in 1979, dropped to 6 per cent. (These figures, which refer to individuals, do not reflect the concentration of wealth, particularly in income-generating forms, in families.) Thus the claim that Thatcherite policies have created a nation of wealth owners is no more than rhetoric. 'Popular' capitalism is as much in the hands of the few as 'unpopular' capitalism.

It is, however, the government's record on poverty that marks the 1980s as the decade of neglect for the weak groups in society. In 1985 the government changed the basis on which it published low-income data; but the Institute of Fiscal Studies used original government data for 1987 to provide the evidence presented here. The sad fact is that the extent of poverty increased considerably between 1979 and 1987.

Table 2.14 uses the Supplementary Benefit definition of poverty. Because so much evidence has been presented to the effect that the level of Supplementary Benefit (or Income Support) is too low even for basic needs, the table provides a range of data for the proportion of people with incomes slightly above the Supplementary Benefit level. It shows that the incidence of poverty was greater in 1987 than in 1979, whichever of these levels is taken to be the poverty line. The table also shows the proportions of people receiving Supplementary Benefit, and although we do not have precise evidence about their incomes, we can assume that at least a small proportion of them had incomes below the Supplementary Benefit level, because of the various rules which disqualify some groups from receiving the standard entitlement and because some others on such benefits simply do

Table 2.14 Proportion of persons in poverty in the UK (per cent)

Cumulative proportions of persons not receiving
Supplementary Benefit with net incomes below
or just above Supplementary Benefit level (%)

Year	*Below SB level*	*Below 110% of SB level*	*Below 120% of SB level*	*Below 140% of SB level*	*Proportion of persons in receipt of SB*
1979	4.0	6.2	9.0	14.4	7.6
1987	5.3	7.7	10.2	14.9	13.5

Source: George and Howards 1991: Table 2.1

not claim all that they are entitled to. Thus at a conservative estimate, we can conclude that in 1987 about 7 per cent of the population had incomes below the Supplementary Benefit level. The risk of poverty, of course, varies between population groups. In terms of incomes below the standard level of social assistance, those above retirement age run the highest risk, followed by the unemployed. Those in full-time employment run the lowest risk even though, because of the size of the group, they make up a large proportion of those in poverty at any one time.

The government's decision to discontinue the publication of data on *Low Income Families*, using the Income Support level as the effective poverty line, makes direct comparison with the post-1987 situation impossible. Instead, the government now publishes *Households Below Average Income*, including figures on the distribution of income among the bottom five deciles of the population. Table 2.15 shows that the real incomes of the bottom half of the population, both before and after housing costs, between 1979 and 1989, increased markedly less than those of the top half. The increase declines as one moves towards the bottom, and indeed the incomes of the bottom decile, after housing costs, actually declined by 6 per cent.

Another way of looking at the changes during the same decade is to consider the proportion of the total national income accruing to the various deciles. The income share going to the bottom half of the population declined between 1979 and 1989: from 33 to 28 per cent before housing costs, and from 32 to 27 per cent after housing costs (DSS 1992: 64).

Table 2.15 Percentage changes in real income by decile group
1979–88/9 in the UK*

Decile 1 Bottom 10%	Decile 2 10–20%	Decile 3 20–30%	Decile 4 30–40%	Decile 5 40–50%	Total population
Income before housing costs					
2	5	9	14	19	28
Income after housing costs					
–6	2	7	14	20	30

Source: DSS 1992: 62, Table A1
Note: * 1988/9 refers to the average figure for the two calendar years

The proportion of the population living in families with
incomes below 50 per cent of the national average rose from 9 per
cent (five million people) in 1979 to 22 per cent (12 million
people) in 1989. The rise was especially high in the case of single
pensioners and single parents with children (DSS 1992: 91). Of
particular concern is the rising incidence of poverty among
children of all economic groups. The number of children living in
households with incomes below 50 per cent of the national average
rose from 1.4 million (10 per cent of all children) in 1979 to 3.1
million (25 per cent) in 1988–9. The increase in the risk of child
poverty suggested by these figures applied even where one or both
parents were in full-time employment; and to the children of both
single and two-parent families (DSS 1992: 99). This cannot but have
detrimental effects, not only on the educational and job careers of
the children, but on the future of economic growth in the country.
If poverty is related to socio-economic group and family status,
however, it is also crucially related to sex. Not only are the
majority of those in poverty women, but also the risk of poverty is
higher for women than for men (Glendinning and Millar 1987).

In the European Community as a whole, the incidence of low
incomes rose only slightly between the mid-1970s and the
mid-1980s. The proportion of persons with incomes below 50 per
cent of average equivalent disposable incomes rose from 12.8 per
cent in the mid-1970s to 13.9 per cent in 1985 (Oppenheim 1990:
121). In the UK, however, the proportion almost doubled – from
6.7 per cent to 12.0 per cent – and this must reflect, to some
extent, the restrictive social security policies pursued by the
government in the 1980s (1990: 121).

So the 1980s saw a marked rise in living standards in the UK – and at the same time considerable increases in inequality and poverty. It was a decade of widening social and regional polarisation which undoubtedly owed much to a variety of public policies designed to have both practical and ideological effects, as well as to secular trends in the British economy and social structure.

'The enterprise culture' and support for welfare

It was an aim of Thatcherism to effect a major shift from the 'welfare' to the 'enterprise' element in British culture, ideology and opinion. Did such a shift take place? This section considers some of the evidence regarding enterprise growth and public opinion.

First, there is no doubt that some of the features of 'enterprise culture' grew during the Thatcher era, whether as a result of Thatcherite policies or otherwise. Two such features are self-employment, to which we shall return, and popular share ownership. As we have remarked, privatisation was an important element of Thatcherite strategy in industrial and welfare terms, and sometimes both at once. The denationalisation of publicly-owned industry was frequently presented as a part of the construction of a 'share-owning democracy'. Whatever the consequences for democracy, there is no doubt that share owning became a much more popular activity during the late 1980s than ever before. The take-off point was the public sale of shares in British Telecom, part of the first of a series of major privatisations. Treasury figures suggest that share ownership rose from about 6 per cent of the adult population in 1984 to about 24 per cent in 1990 (CSO 1991: 96). And, if the purchase of shares in privatised companies introduced people to the habit of share buying, it seems to have led to broader-based activity in the stock-market.

Thus, while only a minority (about a quarter of adults) engage in share owning, and many do so in a very small way, this activity has grown with extraordinary speed since the mid-1980s, has done so among the more affluent and influential groups in the population, and is now an accepted and no longer the rather eccentric activity it once was. While rising standards of living were always likely to bring about such effects to some extent, their scale and timing can be said to represent an achievement for Thatcherism.

There was a scarcely less spectacular rise in self-employment during the Thatcher era. As Daly observes, 'The last decade was a period of unprecedented growth in the number of self-employed people. Between 1981 and 1989, this number grew by 1,248,000 (57 per cent) to 3,425,000' (Daly 1991: 109). These are not primarily captains of industry. Most of the growth (1,010,000) was among the self-employed without employees (1991: 109). Some of these are effectively doing, on new terms, jobs which were previously done by employees – sometimes themselves – rather than initiating entirely new enterprises. Moreover, as Blanch-flower and Oswald (1990) show, much of the increase can be attributed to specific economic factors, in the employment market and elsewhere, at a time of rapid economic change. Nevertheless, again it is a striking phenomenon; no less so for the vulnerability of such small-scale entrepreneurs that was cruelly exposed in the recession of the early 1990s.

Have these and other changes, similarly geared towards giving people a sense of independence and individualism, undermined support for collective activities like welfare policy? There is a grati-fying amount of evidence now available, although its interpretation is not always clear-cut.

Edgell and Duke, on the basis of their Greater Manchester Survey, emphasise the class basis of divisions on, for instance, opinion on cuts in public spending. They found in all groups increasing disapproval of such reductions during the early 1980s, but clear divisions between 'workers' and other groups being maintained (Edgell and Duke 1991). Taylor-Gooby, in the Seventh Report of the British Social Attitudes Survey, concurred with this division but argued that the picture is complicated:

> There is also evidence . . . that better-off people would like to retain access to a substantial private sector operating alongside the welfare state. While in the future there may be tension between support for common state provision and for privileged private services, with 'comfortable Britain' then withdrawing support for common services and opting instead for a two-tier welfare state, such a fracture is not yet in sight.
>
> (Taylor-Gooby 1990: 18–19)

Table 2.16 illustrates the division of opinion to which Taylor-Gooby and so many other commentators refer. It also shows, however, the unambiguous rise in the proportion of res-pondents supporting higher taxes to finance better social services

Table 2.16 Support for UK social spending, 1983 and 1989 compared (per cent)

1983 > 1989 The government should: Total	I/II	III non-manual	III manual	IV/V
Reduce taxes, lower social spending 9 > 3	9 > 2	4 > 2	9 > 4	13 > 3
Keep same as now 54 > 37	59 > 37	59 > 40	56 > 35	49 > 36
Increase taxes, increase social spending 32 > 56	28 > 57	35 > 53	32 > 58	33 > 56

Source: Jowell *et al.* 1990: 21, Table 1.1

in all socio-economic groups during the 1980s.

Less positive altogether on support for the welfare state are Saunders and Harris, the title of whose Social Affairs Unit pamphlet, *Popular Attitudes to State Welfare Services: A Growing Demand for Alternatives?*, reflects their alternative approach to relative preferences between state and private social provision. Essentially, their argument is that the degree of choice which people see as open to them personally is crucial in forming their opinions in respect of private and public provision (Saunders and Harris (n.d.): 27–8). For instance, the existence of conspicuous and potentially accessible alternatives to public provision is much greater in the area of housing than in that of health care, which is dominated by the NHS. The possibility of exit is much greater in housing. Thus dissatisfaction with public housing services is more likely to be expressed in dissatisfaction with the whole sector than is the case in public health care. The choices open to people in their efforts to square their own welfare circles will influence their attitudes to public policy and the squaring of the public welfare circle.

If Saunders and Harris are correct, there is potential for an increase in popular dissatisfaction with the public services towards the year 2000 that is not hinted at in Table 2.16. The impact of Thatcherite policies and changes may become greater over a period of years. However, in the early 1990s the ideological impact of Thatcherism remained unclear. Those who expected a reaction against its values pointed to continued poll reports of public concern about the underfunding of social provision, particularly in health care and schools. Against this, the General Election of 1992, as an opinion poll, suggested that this reaction had limits which kept it a long way short of a counter-revolution. In the case of the Thatcherite attempt to square the welfare circle, it appeared that the jury was still out.

The 1980s, then, was a decade in which policy reflected both a resurgence and a polarisation of ideological commitment. This marked a break with the earlier part of the post-war period, even if that break was more untidy and less clear than some commentators and partisans perceived. Social welfare politics, policy and institutions emerged from the Thatcherite era in a state of flux and uncertainty. This was enhanced by the realisation that the world around them was changing economically, socially and politically at a pace unlikely to slacken as a new millennium approached. In Chapter 3, we seek to describe some of these changes and to identify trends likely to influence the continuing effort to square the welfare circle in the future.

Chapter 3

The welfare circle towards 2000
General trends

Vic George and Stewart Miller

The notion of the affordable welfare state has inevitably meant that 'realism' has overshadowed idealism in recent debates and policies on welfare. But this is usually a one-sided type of realism, concentrating on the cost of welfare programmes. Far less attention is given to the other side of welfare realism: that is, the need that requires to be met. In this chapter we examine the demographic, social and economic changes that should figure on both sides of welfare realism in the 1990s, and their implications both for the need for service provision and for the availability of resources to meet these needs. Such an exercise is full of dangers and it is worth discussing some of them here.

In the first place, it is generally accepted that projections are always likely to be proved wrong however careful the statistical calculations may be. People, communities, markets, and so on, do not always behave according to the expectations of the experts. This is particularly the case with long-term projections when all sorts of variables may unexpectedly intervene to muddy the waters. Projections are also more likely to be proved wrong when dealing with economic rather than purely demographic issues, for the economy of any country today is dependent not only on internal but also on external world factors which are impossible to predict, particularly when the projection covers more than a few years. The second problem involved in the use of projections for social policy is that developments in any one area are influenced by a multiplicity of interacting factors involving the economy, the demography and the family patterns of the country. It is this matrix of interacting factors which is so difficult to construct with any degree of accuracy. Third, there are always the unknown events which emerge to influence social policy developments and which cannot be taken into account in advance projections. Twenty years ago, no one could have foreseen the spread of AIDS and taken it into account in any projections on health-care demand. For these and other reasons, some projections are nothing more than intelligent guesses of future trends and they should be treated as such.

Since the main theme of this book is government ability to square the welfare circle, we begin with those trends which have resource implications. Demographic trends have always featured prominently in these debates and in recent years they have been used to argue for constraints in public expenditure for fear of future government 'overloading' and of generating excessive intergenerational conflict (DHSS 1985). Before looking at demographic trends in any detail, it is worth making the simple but important point that there is no danger of a population explosion in this country either through natural or migration processes. From around 57 million in 1990 the population is projected to grow to 60 million in 2025, after which there will be more deaths than births resulting in a 'natural decrease in population for the first time since 1976' (CSO 1992a: 25). Beginning with the young age groups, we find that the decline in the number of primary school pupils which occurred during the 1970s and the first half of the 1980s reversed itself in the late 1980s with the result that the number of these pupils began to rise and will continue to rise during the 1990s, though they will never reach their pre-1980 level. From around 5 million in 1975, the number declined to about 3.6 million in 1985, then rose to 3.8 million in 1990, and it is projected to rise to 4.1 million by the year 2000 after which it will begin to decline again (Ermisch 1990: 28). Similar trends have occurred in the secondary school population: from around 4.2 million in 1975, the number declined to 3 million in 1990 after which it is projected to rise very slowly to 3.4 million by 2000, continue mildly upwards for five years and then start to decline again. In brief, there will be a slightly higher number of primary and secondary school pupils during the 1990s than during the late 1980s. It is difficult to claim that these mild demographic changes in the primary and secondary school population have any serious resource implications in terms of expenditure, buildings, equipment or teacher numbers. Other factors may, of course, influence the volume of public expenditure in this area during the 1990s.

The decline in the number of 16–19-year-olds which took place during the 1980s will continue in the early 1990s but will reverse itself after that. From 3 million in 1990, the number of persons in this group will decline to 2.7 million in the mid-1990s and then rise to 3 million again by the year 2001 (CSO 1992a: 28). The implications of these figures for higher education are not all that great because entry to higher education does not depend greatly on the size of the relevant age group. To begin with, these demographic trends are even milder in the case of the middle- and higher-income groups which traditionally have been the main sources for higher education students. Also, the numbers and pro-portions of young people passing the required higher education entry qualifications has been rising and, most probably, will continue to rise for a few more years. In addition, the recent emphasis on attracting mature students as well as students from ethnic minority backgrounds will continue and gain momentum in the 1990s. When, in addition, one takes into account the all-party agreement on increasing the number of higher education students, the general conclusion must be that demo-graphic changes in themselves are not of great significance to higher education government spending during the 1990s. Again, other factors will intervene to influence the amount of govern-ment expenditure in this field. The recent government changes in the funding of higher education have meant that the average cost per student in universities has declined and this policy is likely to be retained, irrespective of which political party is in power during the 1990s. This may well counteract the cost implications of the larger number of students who will be in higher education establishments during this period.

Much has been written and many fears have recently been expressed about the ageing of populations in all advanced industrial societies, including the UK. The dominant view which has influenced government policies is that the ageing of the population will mean that in the future governments will find it difficult to finance services and benefits for this age group, and it is therefore prudent for governments to begin to scale down their commitments to this group. Population ageing is the result of two processes: the decline in birth rates and the rise in life expectancy, and so far it has been the former that has exerted the greatest influence in population ageing. Table 3.1 shows the changes in the age structure of the UK population in recent years and the projections for the future. The size of the population group aged 65 years and over increased from 6.2 million in 1961 to 9.1 million in 1991 and it is projected to remain fairly constant up to 2001. After that, current projections are that it will rise gently to 9.7 million in 2011 and then rise more quickly to reach 11.5 million by 2025. The same picture emerges if one looks at this age group as a proportion of the total population: a rise from 11.7 per cent in 1961 to 15.8 per cent in 1991, after which the proportion remains fairly constant until 2011 when it begins to rise more sharply, so that by 2025 it reaches 18.7 per cent of the total population. Some people are particularly alarmed by the rise in the numbers and proportions of the age group aged 80 and over because it is this group that makes a disproportionate demand on the health and personal social services. Each person in this group consumes on average eight times as much of such services as someone aged up to 64 years. Table 3.1 shows that the proportion of this age group has risen twofold between 1961 and 1991, and that it will continue to rise fairly gently so that by 2025 its proportion will be 4.8 per cent of the total population compared to 3.8 in 1991. Other things being equal, it is clear that demographic trends among the older age group will involve a modest rise in public expenditures. What is important for social security expenditure is the number of people above minimum retirement ages – 65 for men and 60 for women. This number is projected to rise from 10.5 million in 1990 to 14.5 million in 2031, a rise of nearly 40 per cent. Though there are some complicating factors, such as the fact that some women may voluntarily decide to work beyond the age of 60 while some men may decide to retire before the age of 65 in greater numbers than at present, these are unlikely to change the general picture. Thus in both social security

Table 3.1 Age structure of the population 1961–2025 (UK)

Year	Under 16		16–64		65–79		80 and over	
	Million	%	Million	%	Million	%	Million	%
1961	13.1	24.8	33.5	63.2	5.2	9.8	1.0	1.9
1991	11.7	20.2	36.8	64.0	6.9	12.0	2.2	3.8
2001	12.6	21.2	37.4	63.2	6.7	11.4	2.5	4.2
2011	12.1	20.1	38.2	63.7	7.0	11.7	2.7	4.5
2025	12.0	19.6	37.5	61.5	8.6	14.1	2.9	4.8

Source: CSO 1992a: 27, Table 1.5

and in health and personal social services, expenditure will need to rise in order to maintain, let alone improve, the standard of present day benefits and services.

The combined number of those below and above working age as a proportion of those in working wage has been referred to as the dependency ratio in society. Clearly, it is a very crude indicator of the ability of a society to bear the economic costs of providing benefits and services to the non-working groups. It is absolutely essential to take into account at least labour participation rates and unemployment rates in these calculations. Falkingham's estimates show that after 1971 'changes in the labour market are more important in influencing dependency than demographic trends' (Falkingham 1989: 225). Therefore, if in the future the proportion of married women in employment rises and the rate of unemployment falls then the standardised dependency ratio, as distinct from the crude demographic dependency ratio, will either fall or remain constant. If the opposite happens, then clearly there may be serious economic consequences for public expenditure unless productivity per person rises substantially to counteract the adverse labour market trends and the effects of demography or sections of the dependent population are enabled to remain in the labour market.

The OECD report on these issues rightly drew attention to the fact that the retired are not a monolithic group, and therefore blanket statements about them are not very helpful in policy terms. In the words of the report: 'While the frail elderly represent a challenge, the active retired constitute a potential resource' (OECD 1988: 19). In a sense this reminds us of the debates concerning the social construction of old age in industrial societies. While there is no good reason to repeat the arguments in detail here, it is worth making the point that retirement ages are not based on any medical or health considerations but rather on industrial and political reasons. This is why they vary so much even among European countries, and why in many of these countries retirement ages have been lowered rather than raised as health standards improved and life expectancy increased. Even if governments find it politically difficult to raise retirement ages, there is no good reason why they should not encourage labour market participation or other forms of work among the young elderly. In brief, the effects of demographic changes on the ability of governments to provide services and benefits are mediated by the influences of other social institutions – 'the nature of retirement, the level of unemployment and the structure of the family' (Taylor-Gooby 1991: 84). Thus labour market factors as well as demographic trends will in reality be the determining influences on public expenditure patterns in the years to come. This is not to deny that governments which wish to reduce the level of public expenditure will not use the demographic card in the future in much the same way as they did in the past. To highlight labour market factors is not to deny the significance of demography – rather it is an attempt to see it in the right perspective. The implications of demography are, perhaps, more worrying for community care services for the very elderly. Wicks quotes figures to show that the proportion of retired people living alone increases with age. Thus, for example, while only 34 per cent of those aged 65 and over live alone, the corresponding proportion of women aged 85 and over is 53 per cent. A high proportion of these either had had no children or had outlived their children. Given the traditional dependence on women for community care and the rising proportion of women in employment, the seriousness of the situation for community care services becomes apparent (Wicks 1987: 158).

We now move on to examine those family trends which are likely to have some bearing on public expenditure during the rest of this decade and beyond. As an institution, the family has always been changing and governments have frequently tried, albeit with little success, to stem the tide of change through mainly negative or restrictive policy measures (Finch 1989). The first clear trend in family patterns is the rise in dissolution rates through either divorce or separation. The number of divorces granted per 1,000 married women rose from a mere 2.5 in 1961 to 13 in 1985 due mainly to the easing of divorce laws. This was most probably accompanied by a smaller decline in separation rates although hard evidence is difficult to come by. When the two trends are combined, it is still the case that family dissolution rates have increased over the years. Moreover, it is difficult to see why this trend will be reversed in the future despite recent government 'pro-family' policies which we will refer to below. The second relevant trend has been the rise and fall of remarriage rates. While only 7 per thousand of divorced men remarried in 1961, the corresponding proportion for 1972 was 13, after which it began to decline so that by 1988 it was a mere 3.5 per thousand. A similar trend was evident for divorced women, though the remarriage figures have always been lower: 4 per thousand in 1961, 7.5 in 1972 and a mere 2.5 in 1988. Even if family dissolution rates remain the same during the 1990s, the fact that remarriage rates are declining means that the number of cohabiting and one-parent families will increase in the future. Indeed, trends in cohabitation rates lend support to this conclusion even though co-habitation applies even more so to never-married women. While only 7 per cent of women marrying in the early 1970s had been cohabiting, the proportion in 1987 was 48 per cent and set to rise even further during the 1990s (Kiernan and Wicks 1990).

The rise in the proportion of one-parent families is the fourth family trend and it is well documented. One-parent families as a proportion of all families with dependent children rose from 8 per cent in 1971 to 19 per cent in 1990 (CSO 1992a: 39). This rise has been the result of two main trends: divorce rates and pre-marital births, though the fundamental causes are to be found in the changing economic position of women in society and the liberal-isation of sexual mores. These fundamental changes in the material and ideological aspects of society explain both the universal rise of one-parent families in all advanced industrial societies and the irreversibility of this trend (Roll 1991). Though a great deal of concern has been expressed concerning the rise of single mothers, it is in fact marriage dissolution that remains the most significant factor in the creation of one-parent families. It is certainly true that the proportion of births outside wedlock rose from 11 per cent of all births in 1979 to 28 per cent in 1990, but an increasing proportion of these births were jointly registered by both parents. In 1971 only 3.8 of these births were jointly registered while in 1990 the proportion was 20 per cent. Thus it is not possible to make projections on future numbers of single mothers solely on evidence of births outside wedlock. The fact is that cohabitation before marriage is becoming almost the norm now, and this inevitably means larger numbers of children born out of wedlock, a high proportion of them to cohabiting couples rather than to single mothers.

The fifth family change which is relevant for our discussion is that the average age of marriage for both men and women has increased by two years during the past two decades. A significant part of this rise is the result of increased cohabitation before marriage, but there is also a more general trend towards older marriages. When this is seen in conjunction with the rising

Table 3.2 Household types in Britain (per cent)

Type of household	1961	1991
One person		
– Under pensionable age	4	11
– Over pensionable age	7	15
Two or more unrelated adults	5	3
One-family households		
Married couples with:		
– No children	26	28
– Dependent children	38	24
– Non-dependent children only	10	8
Lone parent with:		
– Dependent children	2	6
– Non-dependent children only	4	4
Two or more families	3	1
All households	100	100

Source: CSO 1992a: 41, Table 2.4

proportion of young people living away from their parental home, it becomes clear that the number of one-person households among the young has increased with obvious implications for both the volume and type of housing.

These and other family changes are reflected in Table 3.2. The traditional one-family married couple household is not so dominant in Britain as it was 30 years ago, and it will be even less dominant in the future. The proportions of one-person households and of lone-parent households have, on the other hand, increased over the years and will continue to do so in the future. The clear message of all these data on the family is that 'all the key social indicators (are) moving away from the cherished model' (Wicks 1990: 28). It would be far better for all concerned – parents, children and society in general – if governments accepted these family changes and tried to deal with them constructively rather than attempt the futile task of reversing them.

All these trends in household formation, dissolution and reconstitution have various implications for social policy in the future. We saw earlier in the chapter that demographic trends meant that the rise in household formation during the 1980s was to decline during the 1990s and beyond, with obvious implications for housing need. From a high 152,000 new households arising from age distribution changes in 1990, the figure will decline to 43,000 in 2002, rise again to 90,000 in 2012 and decline again to the very low number of 20,000 in 2021 (Ermisch 1990: 38, Figure 15). This decline in household formation, however, will be somewhat counteracted by the trends in marriage and divorce rates and in lone-parent families as well as by the increasing tendency of young people to live away from their parents. On the whole, demographic and family trends will have either a mildly downward or neutral effect on housing need in the future. Economic factors, however, will also influence housing demand either upwards or downwards depending on such obvious factors as unemployment rates, inflation, interest rates, etc. It is this complex matrix of demographic, social and economic factors that will influence housing demand in the future and which is very difficult to map out with any substantial degree of exactitude. It is likely, however, that housing standards will continue to rise and, as a result, housing costs as well – notwithstanding such exceptional falls in house prices as occurred in the early 1990s. The proportion of these housing costs borne by the state in the future will increase if present patterns of government housing subsidy are maintained.

The rise in one-parent families has obvious cost implications for social security. At present, the vast majority of these families rely on benefits and, unless there is a supportive change in government policies, this will continue in the future. The recent government reforms are almost exclusively concerned with forcing fathers to pay towards the maintenance of their children in an effort to both reduce public expenditure and, rather optimistically, to discourage one-parent family formation. It may have some success with the first aim, but it is most unlikely to have any effect on the second simply because the creation of one-parent families is, as we said earlier, the result of very fundamental changes in the economy and ideology of industrial societies. Above all, these reforms will not have any significant effects in the alleviation of one-parent family poverty. The alternative policy of encouraging lone mothers to seek employment can only succeed if adequate and affordable child care arrangements are made, and combined with social security rule changes to allow mothers to keep more of their earnings from work. These measures will reduce poverty, but they may necessitate a rise in public expenditure unless the child care facilities are provided by employers. All in all, it is difficult to escape the conclusion that the rise in one-parent families will exert an upward pressure on public expenditure in the future, particularly if the state of the economy does not improve.

Recent government policy on the family at large has been to shift the financial and human costs of dependence from the state to the family itself. However, as Finch cogently points out, such policies are bound to run into major difficulties, since 'the scope for placing more responsibility on the family is very limited indeed'. If anything, a strong case can be made for 'a redrawing of the boundaries in the opposite direction, with the state taking more of the weight' (Finch 1992: 56).

We now move on to discuss those economic trends that have implications for the resources needed to square the welfare circle. The first of these is the size of the labour force, that is, 'people aged 16 or over who are either in civilian employment or identified by censuses and surveys as looking for work and available to start (whether or not they claim benefits as unemployed)' (Spence 1990: 187). This definition is straightforward for men aged 16–65 because they are expected to be members of the labour force unless they are in higher education, in the armed forces or in prison. However, the definition is more difficult in relation to women because of the cultural expectation that they will care for their children as well as work whenever possible or necessary. Labour force size projections are therefore influenced by the assumptions one makes about married women's participation in the labour market. It is far easier to project the size of the working age population group than the size of the labour force. Bearing these and other qualifications in mind, a recent government study of future labour force trends arrived at the following conclusions.

> In the year 2001, the labour force is projected . . . to be almost 675,000 higher than its mid-1990 level;
> Almost all the projected net increase is among women who are expected to make up 45 per cent of the labour force by 2001;
> The labour force in 2001 will be older than in 1990; a projected rise of 1,625,000 people aged 25–54 more than offsetting the fall of 1,015,000 people aged under 25 in the labour force.
>
> (DE 1991: 269)

Thus on simple numerical grounds, the projection is fairly optimistic. But the reliance on women's labour participation raises questions about the cost of child care provisions and it has implications for the pool of people available to carry out the unpaid caring work for the very elderly and disabled in the family – a task traditionally carried out by married women. It also raises questions about the allocation of work and caring roles between the sexes in society in general which in turn have implications for the size of the labour force. It would be wrong to go on making labour force projections on the assumption that married women will continue indefinitely to carry out the treble role of wage-earner, child-minder and domestic servant.

Closely connected to the issue of the size of the labour force is the question of the quality of labour. It is obviously a more contested issue, for there are differences of opinion on what constitutes quality. However, if one adopts a human capital approach, then the quality of labour in the year 2001 will be better than today, particularly now that women's participation in higher education has caught up with men's. Both the number and proportion of people in the labour force with higher education and training will be higher in 2001 than it is today.

Quantity and quality of labour are only two of the ingredients of what is needed to promote economic growth. Demand for labour is another, and this is far more difficult to project with any degree of accuracy. The depth of the economic recession in 1991 and 1992, however, suggests that unemployment rates will continue to rise throughout 1993 and part of 1994, and that in the 1990s they will be at least as high as those of the 1980s. Thus the decade will be characterised by troughs and peaks in unemployment rates and it is most unlikely that the remaining years of this decade will experience again the low levels of unemployment of the 1970s, let alone the 1960s. Finally, there is the equally important and difficult issue of labour productivity. The 1980s witnessed significant improvements in labour productivity in many sectors of the economy, but there is no way of knowing whether these will extend to other sectors or whether they will be surpassed in the 1990s. In brief, the quantity and quality of labour, the amount of capital investment, the extent of technical innovation, the quality of industrial relations and the nature of foreign competition will determine the rate of economic growth during the 1990s in this country. Though it is not possible to project confidently the rate of GDP growth during the 1990s, a number of forecasts have been made, based on the experience of the 1980s. Anderton and colleagues projected an average rise in annual GDP of 2.5 per cent for 1993–9; only 1.8 per cent annually for the whole decade (Anderton *et al*. 1991: 12). When in 1991 the Policy Studies Institute forecast an annual rate of 2.3 per cent for the next two decades, they did so on the assumption of a number of improvements in industry and in the economy as a whole (Northcott 1991: 344). In view of the fact that the economy actually shrank by 1 per cent per annum during 1991 and 1992 and that projected growth for 1993 is a mere 1 per cent, it seems unlikely that the average for the 1990s will exceed 2.0 per cent per annum. Government projections that the rate of growth of GDP will range from 3.25 to 3.75 per cent during the four years 1993 to 1997 appear at present to border 'on the heroically optimistic' (Hutton 1992). The overall conclusion must therefore be that the resource side of squaring the welfare circle during the 1990s will be problematic, whichever political party is in power. The country is unlikely to witness either the high rates of economic growth or the low levels of unemployment experienced during the post-war period up to the mid-1970s. The signs are that in this the 1990s will be similar to the 1980s.

If the difficulties of squaring the circle purely in terms of needs and resources are becoming greater, so is the task facing a political party wishing to pull off this trick while maintaining its own electability. The changes discussed above have been taking place alongside others which have sometimes threatened to transform the political scene. In particular, the major parties' difficulties in winning parliamentary majorities at general elections have been changing markedly, although, so far, one or other has managed to pull it off on most occasions. The British electoral system, as is well known, tends to favour political parties with a strong class base – working-class Labour and middle-class Conservatives – and to translate national pluralities of votes into absolute majorities of seats in the House of Commons. But the share of the vote going to the two biggest parties – the government party and the chief alternative at any given election – declined from an average of 90 per cent in the decade following the Second World War to an average of about 75 per cent in the 1980s, making this effect less reliable. In 1950, 1951, 1964, 1974 (the second election of that year) and 1992 the system produced only narrow majorities – so narrow in 1974 that it disappeared altogether in the life of the parliament – and in the first election of 1974 no party emerged with an absolute majority. But, whereas in the earlier cases the cause of this result was the extreme closeness of the race between the two big class-based parties, latterly the problem for these parties has been the success of others in the wake of a marked decline in the importance and reliability of class as a determinant of voting behaviour, and a much greater volatility in an electorate apparently more inclined to vote on issues as against traditional allegiances. Moreover, there has been a further marked shift in relative strength away from the Labour Party, triggered by economic, social and political changes.

Heath and his colleagues have attempted to calculate the effects of social change: shifts in the class structure, housing, region, trade union membership, education, ethnicity and religion. Not all of these changes influence voting in the same direction; but all except religious and ethnic change – especially class and housing – are likely to have harmed Labour. It is reckoned that, between 1964 and 1987, these combined social changes probably deprived Labour of 4 per cent of the share of the vote, while adding 2.7 per cent and 1.8 per cent to the shares of the Conservatives and Liberals (or Alliance) respectively (Heath *et al*. 1991: 209). If anything, these figures seem surprisingly low, considering that between 1961 and 1981 those in manual work – the traditional core of Labour support – declined from 57.7 per cent to 45.4 per cent of the economically active population (Heath and McDonald 1987). Nor do they appear to take account of the increasing numbers in the population of elderly people – a group less inclined than others to vote Labour.

But more important for Heath and colleagues are changes in the political system itself, including the increase in the number of centre party candidates, the formation of the (short-lived) Social Democratic Party, the perceived usefulness of tactical voting for third parties, and the apparent ideological polarisation of Conservative and Labour. Of course, these developments themselves may be the results of social change. With the direct social change factors mentioned above, it is calculated that the effect of all this, between 1964 and 1987, was to deprive Labour of 11.6 per cent and the Conservatives of 2.3 per cent of the vote and to give the centre parties an additional 13.8 per cent (Heath *et al*. 1991: 220). Whether or not these analysts' account of the balance of explanatory factors is accurate, the actual shift in voting patterns is not far from their prediction.

What has emerged from these changes is a political system in which a substantial part of the electorate is perceived (by itself and the parties) to be highly sensitive to issues, both of provision and of taxation – the concentration on the National Health Service and income tax in the 1992 election is an illustration of the parties' response to this, and the Conservatives' victory on a 'low tax' ticket, over a Labour Party committed to (rather modest) tax increases to finance service improvements may illustrate the voters' priorities. Over a long period of political continuity and weak opposition, the acclimatisation of the electorate to government committed (however successfully) to reducing personal taxation merely seems to have confirmed the trend of social and economic factors in giving more people a perceived interest in containing taxation and fewer people a perceived interest in maintaining high quality, universal social services across the board.

At the same time, the interest of the class-based parties in courting the centre, where their former supporters either float or now support centrist parties, has become so much greater. In their attempt to capture the middle ground of politics both the main political parties have tried to conceal the contradictions between their social policy commitments and their ability to raise the required resources to finance them. The Conservative Party has now committed itself to maintain and improve standards and coverage of the social services and, at the same time, to reduce even further direct taxation rates – partly for basic ideological reasons and partly because it believes that such low rates inevitably promote productivity and economic growth rates. Yet there is no empirical evidence from either this country or from others that this is the case. The Labour Party has committed itself to even better improvements in all social policy areas and it has been prepared to accept that a small rise in taxation rates for the higher income groups will be necessary for this. On present evidence, neither party can fulfil its promises towards the improvement of the social services. To do that they will have to raise extra resources or reduce expenditure in other areas of government activity. They can raise extra resources through rises in indirect taxation and through more borrowing, but neither of these methods can be sustained for long. Indirect taxes are already high and government borrowing can only be sustained for a few years, for after that it becomes itself a drain on national resources. Moreover, the Maastricht Treaty of 1992 commits EC member governments to restrict their budget deficits (and therefore their borrowing) within severe limits, as a counter-inflationary measure thought essential for the creation of a common EC currency. Redirecting public expenditure from one area to another has always been politically very difficult. The much publicised peace dividend is proving very difficult to achieve. The abolition of mortgage tax allowances, often mentioned as a means of broadening the tax base, has been rejected by both major political parties either for ideological or for electoral reasons or both. Finally, most of the saleable state enterprises have already been privatised, and the potential for further proceeds from this source in the 1990s is extremely limited (Stevens 1992).

In summary, this chapter has shown that needs and demands in the social policy fields will increase during the 1990s while the financial resources necessary to meet these will not rise correspondingly. This conclusion stands whether it is based merely on the evidence from demographic, social and economic trends or on the programmes of the two main parties in the country. Squaring the welfare circle will prove as troublesome in the 1990s as it was in the 1980s.

Chapter 4

Employment
Welfare, work and politics

Sean Glynn

It is generally agreed that the boundaries between economic and social policy are ill-defined and that neither form of policy is superior to the other. Without economic growth social policy objectives are unattainable; without the social services, economic growth suffers and confers no benefits to large sections of the population who contributed towards its attainment. So it is appropriate to begin the discussion of social policy and party political proposals in the 1990s and beyond with the parties' agendas for employment and economic growth.

THE WELFARE–EMPLOYMENT NEXUS

In the future, as in the past, the character and welfare of British society will be determined very largely by the ways in which people are employed or not employed. The importance of employment and the disadvantages of unemployment should need no elaboration since there is a very extensive literature on both (Glynn 1991). While employment, directly or indirectly, is the main source of welfare and unemployment is a major cause of poverty and other social problems, it would be simplistic to construct a crude welfare dichotomy between employment and unemployment. There are many problems in defining and measuring unemployment and there is a lack of consensus regarding definition (Garside 1980). During the past two decades there has been much debate about official definitions which have undergone numerous changes (Johnson 1988: 81–104). Unemployment is only one facet of a complexity of market and institutional arrangements, known as 'the labour market', which have important welfare implications. The state of the labour market affects the welfare of the employed as well as the unemployed because it has implications for job availability, working conditions, wages and taxation. In a slack labour market low pay, underemployment, casualisation and intermittent employment, with related social problems, are more likely to occur. It is clear therefore that the employment situation, as well as actual levels of employment, will be an important influence on welfare needs, attitudes and provisions.

Welfare systems in modern society have been designed to cope with perceived deficiencies in labour markets and, in part, to provide alternatives. This welfare–employment nexus is widely recognised, at least implicitly, by all the main political parties, usually in terms of an implied relationship between growth and welfare. In the past the configuration and success or failure of welfare systems has been largely determined by employment situations (Thane 1982).

Unemployment is a social problem in its own right which demands specific remedies (social security, training, relocation, etc.) and it also affects other areas of social concern and policy (crime, housing, health, etc.). Unemployment relief is a large item in the social security budget and one which tends to move counter-cyclically. A downturn in the level of economic activity will increase the need for unemployment relief while reducing tax revenues. Thus the future of state welfare will be crucially affected by the extent of unemployment and this will be a central feature in the problem of squaring the welfare circle.

Traditionally in Britain the welfare needs of the unemployed have been dealt with through the National Insurance and Income Support schemes which provide benefits on a minimalist needs basis. This two-tier system evolved during the inter-war period when it was concluded that alternatives, such as public works, were likely to be more costly and less efficient (Glynn 1991: 80–91). It continues to be accepted across the political spectrum, and almost without question, that for humanitarian and political reasons, the unemployed must be given welfare support. However, with the sharp rise in unemployment since the 1970s there has been some experimentation with 'workfare' and other solutions for specific, minority categories of unemployed workers, notably young people and long-term unemployed (Digby 1989). Also, the desire to cut costs and reduce unemployment totals has led to some erosion of real and relative benefits and the adoption of methods designed to reduce registration. In the future heavy unemployment, budgetary constraint, and the desire to reduce public expenditure could lead to further developments along these lines. However, at the present time there are no specific party proposals for a radical alteration of the system of unemployment relief.

Since the 1970s Britain has experienced not only rising levels of unemployment but also the development of a looser and more diversified labour market with widening variations in both remuneration and conditions of employment (Gospel 1992: Ch. 8). These changes in the labour market have played an important role in increasing inequalities and giving rise to new welfare needs. In the 1980s the de-regulation of employment, promoted in particular by Lord Young, was designed to extend the 'enterprise culture', liberating employers from 'unnecessary restrictions' and enabling the unemployed to 'price themselves into work' (Young 1985 and 1986). Other policy measures, including trade union legislation, the abolition of wage councils, the rejection of the EC Social Chapter, the encouragement of part-time work and self-employment, have important policy implications. It will be shown below that in economic policy it is in the area of the labour market that the political parties are most markedly opposed (see p. 75).

THE RISE AND FALL OF FULL EMPLOYMENT

Full employment after the Second World War not only made the welfare state possible but also did more to alleviate poverty and other social problems than the welfare system as such. In 1958 Peter Townsend argued that 'full employment and not social insurance has been responsible for the reduction in poverty since the war' (Townsend 1958). Behind post-war full employment lay what was, in terms of historical if not international comparison, rapid economic growth. Growth made welfare expansion a relatively easy achievement in fiscal terms and public expenditure came to be regarded as a vital instrument in promoting social reform and avoiding the return of mass unemployment.

Taking GDP as a proxy for welfare it appears that standards have approximately doubled over the last four decades. GDP per head (in 1980 prices) rose from £2,226 in 1951 to £4,465 in 1983 and real wages showed a similar increase over the same period

(CSO 1987: 15). There is also evidence that the most marked improvements in living standards, compared with pre-war circumstances, were in working-class households (Page 1991). However, the relative shares of different social groups in both pre- and post-tax incomes appear to have remained remarkably constant in the post-war period (O'Higgins 1985). During the post-war boom 'trickle-down' effects were doing relatively little to reduce inequalities in income and wealth. The main form of redistribution which did occur was from the very rich to the relatively rich (Royal Commission on the Distribution of Income and Wealth 1979). In the 1970s the long post-war boom came to an end and, with slower growth and higher unemployment, new attitudes towards welfare began to emerge as shown in Chapter 1. While those on the political left concentrated on the welfare system's inadequacies and injustices, and its failure to promote egalitarianism, it was criticism from the right which had most influence. It began to be argued that government was 'overloaded' and that public expenditure was too high and had become an adverse influence on economic performance (Brittan 1975, 1977; King 1976; Bacon and Eltis 1976). These anti-welfarist views drew heavily upon new classical economics and supply-side views (Hayek 1960, 1978; Friedman 1962; Seldon 1981). At the same time, policy errors and supply-side shocks (OPEC 1 and 2) gave rise to severe inflation and balance of payments problems which placed public expenditure at the centre of debate. Crosland's view that 'the party is over' symbolised the Labour government's acceptance that painful choices had to be made about public spending including welfare. Under the Wilson–Callaghan governments economic necessity and financial crisis appeared to demand sharp cuts in welfare spending and the abandonment of 'full employment'. However, the latter develop- ment made the former intention more difficult to achieve.

In the early 1980s the Thatcher government's stated objective of reducing public spending and taxation was defeated, in large part by the sharp rise in unemployment. There were, of course, reductions in direct taxation and in welfare expenditure, other than that relating to unemployment. As Chapter 5 shows and as Christopher Johnson argues:

> The most significant change was that in benefit for the unemployed, which was the main reason why public

expenditure overshot in the first half of the 1980s, then
undershot in the second half, as unemployment rose to a peak
in 1986, then fell sharply. Because of this, social security rose
from 26 to 30 per cent of expenditure by departments between
1979–80 and 1984–5 but remained at the same proportion in
1989–90. Nearly all of the real increase of 32 per cent occurred
in the earlier period.

(Johnson 1991: 93–4)

In simple terms, economic attitudes moved from the classical view,
which dominated until the end of the inter-war period, to the
Keynesian consensus which emerged in the 1940s and prevailed
until the 1970s, giving way to new classical views (Smith 1987). In
the post-Thatcher era a clearly identifiable new consensus has yet
to emerge. Differences between the political parties on employment issues remain, but policy pronouncements also reflect the
possible emergence of a new consensus on the need to control
inflation at all costs. In the 1950s and 1960s Phillips and Friedman
produced new theories relating to employment and inflation
which became widely accepted (Bleaney 1985). Friedman's
'Natural Rate' concept, which most economists accept and
use, defined a NAIRU (Non-accelerating-inflation-rate-of-unem-
ployment) which, in theory at least, demolished the idea of 'full
employment' as previously conceived (Glynn 1991: vii). There has
always been some degree of vagueness about the exact definition of
'full employment' but in the years between 1940 and 1970 it came
to mean, in reality, unemployment at 2 per cent or less. According
to G.D.N. Worswick there are no problems regarding definition:

By full employment, I mean a state of affairs in which everyone
who wants to work, can. Much work is arduous and repetitive;
and it is not always easy to see it in the role of liberator. But can
anyone deny the role which the possibility of employment
outside the home has played during this century in advancing
the status and extending the freedom of women? Someone who
is able and willing to work, but is unable to find a job, is being
denied a basic human right in a civilised society.

(Worswick 1991: 4)

Many economists would point out that the above definition makes
no reference to wages and most would agree that if the
unemployment level is pushed below the 'natural rate' it will have

inflationary consequences. It appears that the former concept and aim of 'full employment' has gone and with it went the political axiom that no government could survive a substantial increase in unemployment. Concern about unemployment has been replaced by the aim of 'beating inflation' and since 1979 unemployment has become, in effect, the principal means of achieving this aim. Britain has moved from a system in which the economy was managed in order to support the social aims and mechanics of the welfare state including 'full employment' to a situation in which, for political and economic reasons, this is no longer deemed to be possible or desirable.

By the 1980s most economists, including those who still called themselves 'Keynesians', accepted the 'natural rate' hypothesis and the new economic 'realism' which held that 'full employment' in the old sense was simply an impossible aim. The emergence, and political success, of 'Reaganism' in America and 'Thatcherism' in Britain promoted a move towards a new post-Keynesian political orthodoxy which was clearly established by the late 1980s (Bleaney 1985; Smith 1987). This change in attitudes is clearly reflected in the policies of the main political parties which indicate a major change in the intellectual and political climate. By the early 1990s no political party was prepared to advocate a return to 'full employment'.

During the past two decades economics has increasingly tended to retreat into econometric abstractions and has been conspicuously unsuccessful in providing solutions to real world problems. Meanwhile, social theorists have failed to suggest ways in which the more important social aims can be reconciled with perceived economic realities. While some economists are pre-pared to advocate ways of reducing unemployment, this is normally through an ingenious searching for loopholes in the current orthodoxy (Davies 1985; Layard 1986). Worswick, in advocating a return to 'full employment', is a major exception (Worswick 1991). Bodies which lobby and campaign against unemployment such as the Employment Institute and the Campaign for Work do not represent a radical intellectual alternative. John Grieve Smith is one of a few who have attempted to argue a full and positive case for 'full employment' outside the prevailing orthodoxy (Smith 1992). Social theorists have failed to seize upon the irony and adverse effects of a set of beliefs which argues in favour of 'choice' while denying to so many the most important choice of all – employment. Economists have ignored the positive case for full employment and have provided a rationale for the acceptance of mass unemployment and its consequences.

For many years opinion polls have shown that unemployment is a leading issue of public concern, but its influence on voting behaviour is less evident. The 1980s have shown that it is possible for governments to survive mass unemployment. While unemployment continues to be a major issue of debate and concern, controlling inflation has become the priority. The political record of the last two decades suggests that inflation may be less politically acceptable than unemployment. While many economists argue that only unanticipated inflation is harmful, politicians sense that inflation gives rise to serious discontent, causes severe adjustment problems and may, if not controlled, threaten the economic and social system. Sadly, during the past two decades non-deflationary means of restraining inflation have either been deemed unsuccessful or have not been tried. As a result, British society has paid an enormous price in terms of jobs lost, businesses ruined and growth lost. At the same time, the hidden costs of unemployment in terms of wasted potential, loss of choice, decreasing job satisfaction and deteriorating conditions of work have been largely ignored, as have many of the less direct welfare costs. It is widely accepted that Britain's most pressing economic need is to improve productivity through investment in human capital and improvement in work-force quality. However, in conditions of heavy unemployment both individual and employer incentives to invest in and undertake training are likely to remain deficient (Glynn and Gospel 1993). While all the political parties give a good deal of attention to training, they do so largely in supply-side terms and give insufficient attention to the demand-side of the labour market.

FUTURE PROSPECTS FOR EMPLOYMENT

The work-force will continue to grow absolutely but will decline proportionately in the 1990s as the dependency ratio increases (the work-force includes the unemployed). However, none of these projected demographic changes are dramatic, as Chapter 3 showed. The setting of new retirement ages for state pension purposes could have a more significant effect on dependency ratios. At the lower end of the age scale the projected expansion in age cohorts should coincide with rising participation in higher education and training and this may ease labour market entry problems, but much will depend on levels of economic activity.

Up to 1997 the labour force will grow very slowly, unlike the early 1980s. Also, the entry of married women into the work-force has been largely completed. The 1990s recession had its main impact in the south-east and the fastest rise in unemployment was in the 25–35 age group. Again, this is in marked contrast to the 1980s recession which left groups of older, mainly industrial unemployed, trapped in depressed areas outside the south-east. With a more flexible work-force, more dependent on tertiary activity, the unemployment hangover of the 1990s recession could be less severe than in the 1980s.

The trends of declining male and rising female participation seem likely to continue at slower rates. Trends towards increasing part-time work, especially for females, are likely to continue but growth in self-employment may be less rapid. The work-force is now divided between the secondary or manufacturing sector (one-fifth) and the tertiary or service sector (four-fifths) with less than 2 per cent in agriculture. Since the mid-1970s the manufacturing work-force has declined relatively and absolutely and there has been concern about this 'de-industrialisation' of the work-force (Bazen and Thirlwall 1989; Blackaby 1979). It may seem reasonable to expect this trend to continue in future given the potential for introducing labour-saving technology in manufacturing and the lack of competitiveness in British industry. However, the main form of technical change influencing employment in the immediate future may be in information technology, which could affect office work more than manufacturing industry. Clearly this would have important implications for female employment, in particular. In the USA, Leontieff and Duchin predict a sharp decline in the office labour force as a result of automation and a similar development may be anticipated in Britain (Leontieff and Duchin 1985). A declining demand for labour in manufacturing and office work suggests an increasing reliance on the more labour-intensive services including distribution and leisure. Clearly there will be an increasing need for a more flexible labour force and both training and retraining will have an important role. Recent cuts in public sector training and education budgets seem set to continue and the effectiveness of TECs remains to be seen.

Future employment levels and unemployment will depend most heavily upon economic circumstances and general levels of economic activity. In simple terms, the amount of unemployment will be determined by the relationship between output, labour productivity and the size of the work-force. If productivity continues to grow at an average long-run rate of about 2.5 per cent per annum, as it did in the 1980s, and the work-force grows 0.5 per cent per annum, then growth in output must be at least 3 per cent per annum in order to prevent an increase in unemployment. Britain's average long-run rate of growth in economic output since 1945 has been 2.6 per cent per annum. However, this conceals a tendency towards lower growth since the early 1970s. Since then the economy has entered three recessions (the mid-1970s, the early 1980s and the early 1990s), with progressively higher levels of unemployment. After each recession so far, unemployment has failed to return to the pre-recession level and falls in unemployment have lagged behind recovery. Exact historical comparisons of unemployment levels are not possible because of changes in the official data (Glynn 1991: Ch.11). In January 1992, the independent Unemployment Unit estimated that, on the pre-revised basis, unemployment was 3.7 million against an official figure of 2.6 million, or 9.2 per cent. Levels of employment during the remainder of the 1990s will depend largely on what growth rates can be achieved. It seems probable that growth will be constrained by both economic capacity and economic policy. Many economists anticipate that unemployment will remain above 2.5 million, on the official figures, for the rest of the 1990s.

It is generally accepted that Britain's future will be crucially affected by developments in the European Community (EC). In economic terms the EC is associated with product market extension and, in theory at least, greater competition in non-primary markets, the increasing multinationalisation of business, integration of financial markets and fiscal and monetary integration on stricter lines. The EC also has a political and social programme which aims at freer movement of labour and improved living and working conditions (but not full employment). Progress towards the regulation of labour market activities has been slow and second order, and Britain has been notoriously unenthusiastic. Nevertheless, there has been gradual movement towards an EC labour market system through statutes, treaties, regulations, directions, recommendations, court decisions and other mechanisms. The main policy measures to bring about social objectives are contained in the Charter of Fundamental Rights of Workers 1989 (the Social Charter) and its related Action Programme, and the Social Protocol of the Maastricht Treaty, 1991, which Britain did not accept. Quite clearly there is open conflict between the social objectives of the EC and the Conservative approach to the labour market. It remains to be seen how this conflict will be resolved. At the same time, the economic and financial implications of closer European integration seem likely to be more important for British workers than the Social Charter.

Policy constraints on growth continue to arise because of Britain's tendency towards higher inflation than competitor economies; the failure to find a remedy for this other than unemployment; a high propensity to import, and a balance of payments weakness. By the end of 1991 it was widely believed that Britain had entered the broad band of the ERM at too high a parity and that this compounded these problems. It seemed possible that Britain's experience of the ERM in the 1990s, even assuming an inevitable devaluation, would echo that of France in the 1980s: the adjustment to European inflation levels might involve a lengthy period of economic restraint and high unemployment. Then the summer of 1992 saw a crisis which forced sterling's departure from the ERM and subsequent devaluation. The future became if anything less easy to predict but many commentators, influenced by continuing recession in Britain and adverse international trends, immediately revised predictions of future unemployment levels upwards, to 3.5 million by the end of 1993 and a plateau of 3 million for much of the 1990s. On the other hand the removal of the monetary restrictions of the ERM, and the easing of inflationary pressures through recession, provide possibilities for more expansionist policies including lower interest rates and a larger budget deficit. By the autumn of 1992 the future of European integration and Britain's likely role in it had become much more uncertain. Also, there were signs of important changes in economic opinion. Economic policies for the rest of the 1990s could be less restrictive than previously anticipated.

Since 1945 Britain has experienced lower growth rates than most other industrial economies (Crafts and Woodward 1991: Ch. 9). While there are many different interpretations of Britain's relative economic decline there is general agreement that successive governments have been obliged to restrain growth because of weakness on external account. During each of the past three decades there have been attempts to nudge the economy on to a higher growth and productivity path. These include the Maudling 'dash for growth' in the 1960s; the 'Heath–Barber boom' of the early 1970s and the 'Lawson boom' of the late 1980s (Cairncross 1992). Each of these ventures encountered resource constraints and ran into inflation and balance of payments problems. In each case, after short bursts of growth, the economy had to be sharply reined back by the introduction of deflationary measures. It is now clear that the much vaunted 'economic miracle' of the 1980s was a mirage and the economy's funda-mental economic weaknesses remain all too apparent (Riddell 1991). In the early 1990s a severely depressed economy continued to have a relatively high rate of inflation, in terms of international comparison, and a heavy current account deficit. Constrained growth and heavy unemployment are likely to continue through the 1990s but much depends on the evolution of exchange rate policy and the willingness to use other policy measures to alleviate unemployment.

The Conservatives have been criticised for excessive reliance on monetary policy, in particular high interest rates. The other parties would be more inclined to use fiscal measures, although Maastricht, together with some pre-election promises and a PSBR of £28 billion and rising, imply limited flexibility. All the main political parties appeared to favour membership of the ERM and the Conservatives were criticised for their delayed decision to join. The Major government used Maastricht to keep open an option on the single European currency and Labour also has declined to make a total commitment. Before September 1992 the issue of parity, for obvious reasons, was not openly discussed, but in all parties there appeared to be some support for devaluation through realignment and some for withdrawal from the ERM. However, across most of the political spectrum there appears to be a general acceptance that Britain's economic future is bound up with Europe and that this is inevitable and might as well be accepted. Many would admit that this may involve economic and social hardships as Britain attempts to overcome its inflation, balance of payments and productivity problems. An analogy, perhaps unfortunate, often used is that of a man on a ship which is destined to hit the rocks. The choice is between jumping into the sea, at the risk of drowning, or staying on board and hoping to survive the impact. Britain's three main political parties have decided to stay on board in the hope of reaching shore relatively unscathed.

In May 1992, the National Institute of Economic and Social Research, in its quarterly survey, predicted that Britain faced a prospect of mass unemployment lasting until the next century. The official unemployed total was predicted to reach three million in the summer of 1993 and to remain at or near that level for the remainder of the decade. The Institute pointed out that the scope for fiscal expansion was limited by the state of the public finances and ERM membership precluded monetary expansion or currency devaluation (NIESR 1992). With devaluation and departure from the ERM, some of these restrictions no longer apply. However, much depends on the effects of devaluation, and the extent to which the possibilities for relatively expansionary policies are utilised. Inflation and balance of payments problems will remain and restrict the scope for expansionist measures, especially if Britain resolves to rejoin the ERM and ratifies the Maastricht Treaty. In any case, British growth is likely to be constrained by depleted and inadequate industrial capacity and a tendency towards higher inflation than elsewhere.

If growth is unlikely to be sufficient to solve employment problems and monetary and fiscal policies are constrained, then the only way to reduce unemployment is through active labour market measures, both on the demand side – employment-creation schemes – and on the supply side – education, training and other measures. In a situation of constrained growth, active labour market measures will have to carry a very heavy burden, and none of the main political parties seems to be sufficiently aware of this fact. Nor is there sufficient awareness of the need to find alternative ways of dealing with inflation, or of tackling the balance of payments problem through enhanced industrial capacity.

EMPLOYMENT POLICY AND THE POLITICAL PARTIES

During the 1980s there were important changes in Labour Party policy including dramatic reversals on nationalisation, council house sales, trade union reform and nuclear weapons. On economic policy, Labour entered 1992 with a serious credibility gap regarding its capacity to manage the economy, and the Party leader was accused of being less than convincing on economic matters. While Labour sought to campaign on growth and employment issues it found itself quite often on the defensive as its opponents argued that Labour policies would raise rather than lower unemployment.

For a clear statement of Labour Party policy on employment it is possible to rely heavily on the Policy Review of the late 1980s (Labour Party 1988). This commenced after Labour's third consecutive election defeat in 1987, during the 'triumphalist' phase of Thatcherism. Not surprisingly the review displays an ambivalence between traditional Labour values and the new economic perceptions. However, the review is a more radical document than Labour's public pronouncements in recent years suggest. It has been argued that Labour moved in the direction of market economics in the late 1980s just at the wrong time. As a result, in the early 1990s it was caught on the wrong foot as the economy slid into the longest recession since the 1930s and market economics began to come under attack.

In the 1987 election, Labour made unemployment an issue but avoided any promise of a return to 'full employment'. The manifesto, *Labour Will Win* (Labour Party 1987), stated: 'We must as a priority tackle the immediate tragedy and waste of unemployment'. Labour's pledge to cut unemployment by one million in two years was probably realistic but it may not have been viewed in this way by the electorate. Employment policy was examined by the Policy Review Group and the final report committed Labour to 'a fully-employed economy in which everyone of working age has the opportunity to take paid work'. It continued, 'It is a long time since full employment was the objective of government, so long that as a goal it may seem unrealistic. However, as we explain in this report, it is a goal that can be achieved' (Labour Party 1988: 17). This aspect of Labour policy has not been much emphasised by Labour front-benchers, and most members of the public in the early 1990s would have been surprised to hear that Labour was committed to full employment, as defined in the above quotation, and believed that this could be achieved.

More recent literature has been produced against a background of sharply rising unemployment, and full employment is less often mentioned. In the publication *Opportunity Britain: Labour's better way for the 1990s* it is predicted that under present policies unemployment will rise above three million again in 1993 before 'bottoming out' at higher levels in the 1990s than in the 1980s (Labour Party 1991b: 4–5). In order to deal with unemployment there is emphasis on training, investment and growth. The same publication states that the official figures are 'fiddled' (1991b: 8) and, under the heading 'cutting unemployment', it mentions the following measures: sustained and steady growth, regional policies, training, careers advice, and special temporary employment measures. The last of these involved a special programme which would offer three days' work per week, plus training and time for job-seeking, to unemployed workers.

In addition to this, however, Labour is committed to work-force change:

> If people are to make the greatest possible contribution to the success of their enterprise they need work which makes good use of their abilities, which pays a decent wage, offers reasonable security and working conditions and provides opportunities for training and retraining.
>
> (Labour Party 1988: 17)

With these aims in mind Labour proposed to promote genuine equal opportunities, and to find ways to increase investment in education and training: 'Our economy must transform itself into a knowledge-based economy: an economy which depends on people's intelligence, adaptability and co-operation' (1988: 18). They proposed to promote effective trade unions and to establish worker rights in line with the EC Social Charter. Also, to offer public service traineeships to all the unemployed and to 'integrate' academic and vocational training for 16–19-year-olds.

These commitments, presented to the Party Conference in 1988, reflect, on the one hand, the Party's long-standing commitments, for example, to the trade unions and to the cause of equal opportunities; on the other hand, they indicate an awareness of the classical revival in economics. But Keynesian reflation is not ruled out: 'Full employment will not come about merely through the manipulation of aggregate demand. Everyone must have the opportunity to acquire the skills and wherewithal to adapt' (Labour Party 1988: 4). There are elements of uncertainty in the precise meaning of 'full employment' when it is suggested that training and early retirement 'are factors to be taken into account in a modern definition of full employment in a free society' (1988: 4). Labour has attempted to echo the arguments of those economic analysts and commentators who suggest that the industrial future lies in terms of more intensive exploitation of human capital. They argue that Britain should try to develop a more flexible and sophisticated work-force which is well paid and protected in terms of rights in employment They suggest that 'Economic change and social justice must advance together, aided by a framework of individual rights and collective organisation' (1988: 17). The Policy Review sets out a detailed programme for training, both for the employed and the unemployed. Labour accuses the Conservatives of attempting to move in the opposite direction by seeking a national economic advantage in terms of a low paid, unorganised and unprotected labour force. The Conservatives counter these arguments by suggesting that interference in the labour market inhibits enterprise and employment. They suggest, for example, that the introduction of a minimum wage would destroy jobs on a substantial scale. The Policy Review shows a clear understanding of the magnitude of the problem which a Labour government committed to full employment would face. It is also clear about the costs of unemployment:

> Although unemployment is unevenly spread over areas, ages, skill groups and on women, people with disabilities and racial minorities, the repercussions of mass unemployment are felt by everyone. The growth of poverty and the restriction of job prospects for new generations of workers are a corrosive influence on society and a costly drain on the economy. As many other countries recognise, the costs of unemployment far outweigh the expense of creating jobs.
>
> (Labour Party 1988: 26)

Labour plans a co-ordinated attack on unemployment involving employers, trade unions and local authorities. For the unemployed they propose a training package as well as higher benefits and relaxation of the rules relating to voluntary work and study.

The employment section of the Policy Review is an impressive programme, well argued and detailed. On paper, the programme is humanitarian while also addressing some basic weaknesses in the British economy. Two major doubts arise, however. First, the intended input from central government hardly seems sufficient to support a policy of full employment; and second, it is not clear how inflation would be controlled.

The Labour Party Manifesto of 1992 was entitled *It's Time to Get Britain Working Again* and its main emphasis was on economic recovery. Under the heading 'Action for jobs', stress was placed on housing investment and the pledge to establish a work programme was reiterated. A swift reduction in unemployment was promised under the National Recovery Programme and it was suggested that growth and training were the essential avenues to higher employment (Labour Party 1992b: 12). The need for co-ordinated growth in Europe was also mentioned. The previous emphasis on training, for both the employed and the unemployed, was reiterated with the aim that 'Britain's future must be high skill, high wage and high tech' (1992b: 13) and that employees should have fair treatment at work under the European Social Chapter. In brief, Labour's manifesto proposals on employment and related issues were in line with the previous policy pronouncements outlined above. But full employment was not pledged and there was little to suggest that if Labour had won the election a determined and direct assault on unemployment would have resulted. In the Labour leadership elections which followed the general election defeat Bryan Gould, the unsuccessful candidate, suggested in a BBC radio interview that it was time for Labour to 'reiterate' its commitment to 'full employment'.

It is frequently observed that the Liberal Democrats need not fear the implications of their policy pronouncements since they are very unlikely to assume office. This was less true in the early part of 1992 than in previous pre-election periods. In terms of name at least, the Party was a relatively new formation still seeking a clear policy stance as well as an elusive and disappearing middle ground. Policy pronouncements still reflect the lingering influence of David Owen and the idea of the 'social market' has remained. There is little evidence that the Liberal Democrats are committed to 'full employment' in any recognisable form but their literature shows a determination to reduce unemployment and a clear appreciation of the costs of unemployment both to society and the individual. Liberal Democratic documents emphasise the links between different areas of policy: 'Economic, educational and environmental policies are thus the building blocks of our future, and European union and electoral and constitutional reform the essential foundations' (Liberal Democrats: n.d.).

The Party's working group on economic policy is clearly well informed about recent developments in economic theory, including the rational expectations hypothesis. They 'take seriously the argument that markets may anticipate the effects of government policies and thereby limit their effectiveness' (Liberal Democrats 1991a). The solution to this problem lies 'through the adoption of simple, publicly announced policy guidelines or "rules" for government's macro economic management'. They also advocated entry of sterling into the narrow band of the ERM as soon as possible (no mention of parity, but devaluation was rejected), rapid progress towards Economic and Monetary Union, including a single currency and an independent central bank, plus 'an independent UK central bank charged with ensuring price stability, and an active fiscal policy' (1991a: 30). Specific measures to reduce unemployment are both demand- and supply-side and include more training, spending on infrastructure, energy-conservation projects and housing, plus a shift of taxation from employers' National Insurance towards 'taxes on resources' (1991a: 30). Specific proposals on the labour market include substantial investment in education and training (financed by a 1p rise in the basic rate of income tax) and a requirement on employers to release 16–18-year-olds for two days per week for training and/or education; a reformed system of TECs and LECs; and a Training Levy of 2 per cent on payrolls and the extension of profit sharing (1991a: 30).

Liberal Democrat policy puts some emphasis on demand-side measures while being very critical of Conservative policies. The YTS schemes are described as being 'little more than a source of cheap labour for private enterprise', and emphasis is placed on long-term training needs (Liberal Democrats 1991d). Late in 1991 as unemployment rose, Liberal Democrat policy pronouncements began to take a more interventionist turn. In *The Price of Unemployment* it was claimed that 'Unemployment is out of control'. Levels of three million by March 1992 were predicted and it was suggested that 'the longer term outlook is equally bleak' (1991c: 1). This document sets out to draw up an 'initial quantification' of the price of unemployment. Clear links between unemployment and poverty are established and it is suggested that over 50 per cent of the poorest families were affected by unemployment.

Not only has the value of unemployment and related benefits been cut in real terms since 1979 by around 5 per cent, but the benefit system itself has become more restrictive in its regulations and starved of resources for its administrative efficiency. The government's policy for much of the late 1980s seemed to be to blame the unemployed for being out of work and penalise them through their social security policies.

(Liberal Democrats 1991c: 1)

Unemployment is linked to the problems of homelessness, ill-health, early deaths, suicides and nutritional deficiencies. The direct annual Exchequer cost per unemployed person is estimated at £8,082 and it is pointed out that for each 100,000 rise in unemployment, social security payments are expected to increase by £305 million. In July 1991, the Liberal Democrats produced a programme to reduce unemployment (Liberal Democrats 1991b). This put forward 'sensible, affordable measures' to create 'jobs, places and secondees' totalling 'up to 396,500' through a total (gross) expenditure of £33 billion. A range of measures was highlighted including a Local Employment Initiative, releasing and making available additional funds to local authorities; an Energy Employment Scheme involving energy conservation measures; an increase in training funds for TECs; increased support for secondments; additional enterprise allowances; and measures to reduce late payment of debts (unspecified). All of these proposals were in keeping with previously stated Liberal policies and there was renewed emphasis on the importance of an independent central bank. A similar but more expansive package was promulgated in February 1992. This involved expanding the PSBR by £6 billion. The Liberal election manifesto, *Changing Britain for Good*, was firmly social market in approach, stressing the need for a more efficient economy but with an important regulatory role for government. Thus the Liberals committed themselves to an 'emergency programme of investment in the infrastructure and in public works . . . reducing unemployment by 600,000 over the next two years' (Liberal Democrats 1992: 18). In view of the anticipated rise in unemployment this was perhaps a modest proposal, and it was coupled with a pledge to give the Bank of England independent responsibility for monetary policy and to enter the narrow band of the ERM. The only other specific provisions for the unemployed related to education and training (1992: 20). Tackling unemployment was not a major feature of the manifesto and the implications for employment of other policy proposals were ignored. For example, there was considerable stress on the need for new environmentalist policies, including the need to re-define GDP (1992: 28), but the labour market effects, potentially enormous, were ignored. Apart from its 'emergency programme' and provisions for education and training the Liberal Democrats did not offer any specific measures for confronting unemployment directly. They shared a commitment with the other parties to an improved economy in which employment might be higher.

Both the main opposition parties sought to identify the Conservative Party with unemployment and this was reminiscent of an earlier phase in post-war history. Much was made of John Major's comment, 'If it isn't hurting it's not working', and Norman Lamont's unfortunate statement, 'Rising unemployment and the recession have been the price that we have had to pay to get inflation down. That price is well worth paying' (Hansard, 16 May 1991). Like the other parties, the Conservatives were ill-prepared for the sharp escalation of unemployment in 1991–2. At the beginning of 1990, Michael Howard claimed: 'we have moved into the 1990s enjoying the largest fall in unemployment on record' (Conservative Party 1990: 59). In the months that followed, the Employment Secretary enhanced his reputation as a barrister who made the best of a bad brief. In the face of rising unemployment ministers argued that this was part of 'a worldwide phenomenon' and that the only way to tackle the problem was to 'defeat inflation' (1990: 7): 'The battle against inflation is crucial to long-term job prospects; inflation is the mother and father of unemployment' (1990: 3). The distinction between 'long-term jobs' and other kinds of employment remained both unclear and controversial as did the implication that, in order to avoid un-employment, it was necessary to defeat inflation by having increased unemployment. The Conservative measures dealing directly with unemployment were listed as including: A guarantee of training to every 16 and 17 year old unemployed school leaver; employment training for the long-term unemployed; Job Clubs offering free job-hunting and advice; the Job-Interview Guarantee and TECs (1990: 4–6).

Early in 1992, in an atmosphere of growing concern over rising unemployment, Central Office felt obliged to issue a new list of measures to tackle unemployment. Despite this move, policy remained very much as before. Stress was placed on 'job creation' since 1983, the industrial relations 'reforms' which 'made job creation possible' (Conservative Party 1990: 60). In March 1989, a network of TECs (about 100) was announced and it was claimed that the UK had 'a far higher proportion of people in work than almost any other EC country' (1990: 68). The 1991 Campaign Guide accused Labour of ending post-war 'full employment' in the mid-1970s and claimed:

> The causes of this substantial increase in unemployment were manifold: rampant inflation; high wage costs and low investment; heavy taxation and regulations on business; the excessive power of the trade unions; and a fundamental neglect of the country's training needs.
>
> (Conservative Party n.d.: 128)

The Guide goes on to claim that the main reasons why 'it proved so difficult to bring unemployment down' in the 1980s were because of an increase in school-leavers and more women entering the labour market. Government strategy for employment is said to contain three key elements: first, 'sound economic policies'; second, the removal of 'barriers to job creation' such as employment protection laws; and third, 'increased training'.

In a section devoted specifically to unemployment it is claimed (wrongly) that 'only one significant change has been made' to the unemployment figures (the ending of registration). The 'basic link' between pay and jobs is stressed, as is the need for a slower rise in real wages, and the fallacy of incomes policies which have 'always failed to work'. Government action to reform the labour market has involved the removal of 'unnecessary restrictions' such as Wages Councils and the Dock Labour Scheme. Local pay bargaining and profit-related pay are recommended (p. 133). Under the heading 'Help for the Unemployed' the Guide mentions 'reforms' in the Employment Service, Job clubs, the Job Interview Guarantee, Restart, Youth Training, Employment Training, Job share, and help for the disabled (pp. 135–6). The work of 'Claimant Advisors' in preventing fraud is also mentioned. Deindustrialisation is dismissed rather lightly and it is suggested that a new attitude towards manufacturing industry is required (p. 137): 'Productivity and profitability are better indicators of its success than are its levels of employment'. Under training it is claimed:

For far too long Britain gave insufficient attention to training the key elements in the work-force. This Government has taken decisive action to correct that error. It has introduced the most ambitious and successful training programme the country has ever seen.

(Conservative Party n.d.: 137)

Quite clearly these claims contain a good deal of political rhetoric as well as cynicism. Conservative literature has sought to match or to negate the employment proposals of other parties and it has probably achieved some success. The Conservative manifesto, *The Best Future for Britain* (Conservative Party 1992), was attacked on publication for its total lack of comment on the unemployment problem and the irony of offering 'choice' to the unemployed. Even in the section on education and training, entitled 'Opportunity for All', any mention of unemployment was carefully avoided, although it was clear by implication that most of the 'training' provisions were aimed at the unemployed. Similarly, the section on social services made no mention of the unemployed, apart from a suggestion that the social security system in the past had created 'barriers to work' (1992: 29). Clearly the Conservatives concluded that they had nothing to gain, and possibly much to lose, in raising the unemployment issue. They chose, therefore, to ignore it. In effect, this was a more extreme form of the strategy adopted by the other two parties, which also chose to play down the issue in comparison with previous elections. During the general election of 1992 unemployment was not a major issue, except as an aspect of economic recession. No party offered a convincing programme for what was confidently expected to be a long-term problem. Clearly, in the long run Keynes was very dead, and anything approximating to full employment was not on the agenda.

TOWARDS 2000

The literature of the three main political parties on the subject of employment (and unemployment) displays ostensible similarities and some underlying differences. All three parties emphasise the need to control inflation, without producing a clear and unambiguous strategy for doing so. Labour's hidden agenda might include an incomes policy and a reversion to some form of corporatism, while the other two parties, in their heart of hearts, might accept that unemployment was in the final analysis their main weapon against inflation. It is clear that all three parties were caught out by the sharp rise in unemployment in 1991–2 as the recession deepened and lengthened. No party had a programme for employment creation on a sufficient scale to tackle the problem in the short run. All had unconvincing long-term proposals for unemployment which placed a heavy emphasis on training and other supply-side measures, but the demand-side was ignored or heavily neglected (Glynn and Gospel 1993). Policy statements from all three parties reflected an acceptance of the limitations of economic policy and governmental influence and all accept further limits in terms of links with Europe. They also accept that market forces are, and should be, the major determining influence on income distribution. This in particular may be Margaret Thatcher's most important legacy. The welfare ideal has been replaced by a market ideology which is labelled 'realism'.

Although unemployment has been used as the main weapon for dealing with inflation, recent experience suggests that it is a clumsy and damaging device which tends in British circumstances not to be very effective. Economists have argued that many of the unemployed are effectively outside the labour market and therefore have no influence on the process of wage-determination (Layard 1986). In the 1980s sharp increases in real wages continued through heavy unemployment and despite a weakened trade union movement. Recent experience also suggests that unemployment may be cumulative and that, once created, it tends to linger even when the economy recovers.

There are grounds for believing that British economic growth during the 1990s will be constrained by both circumstances and policy so that a return to full employment is very unlikely. Most economists doubt that unemployment will fall much below 2.5 million on the official count. Growth limits imply that beyond cyclical recovery there will be a need for active labour market measures which emphasise demand as well as supply. In placing emphasis on supply the political parties lack effective policies for dealing with unemployment. All the parties recognise the need for more training but policies remain biased towards the supply-side. In effect, there appears to be an implicit faith that supply creates its own demand. This is a questionable belief at a time when most of what is called training is, in effect, unemployment relief. Effective training must be based upon a sound education system since training without education is a nonsense. In a slack labour market both personal and employer incentives for more training are likely to remain deficient. The only way to establish fully effective training incentives is through job availability. Full employment in the old sense is no longer a priority for the political parties, although some of them openly recognise the heavy costs of unemployment. While unemployment continues to be viewed as 'a price worth paying' in order to control inflation, any return to full employment is out of the question. Alternative ways of controlling inflation are not being sought, essentially for political reasons.

Countries which have been most successful in limiting inflation appear to have done so by moving in one of two directions: either they do so on the basis of largely unregulated free market systems, as in the United States, or, like Germany, they have well-developed corporatist arrangements through which employers, trade unions and government co-operate to control wage–price rises. Britain may have fallen between the two although, in the 1980s, there was a determined attempt to adopt the American model. In the process, corporatist structures and tendencies were largely destroyed. If Britain is to become a successful member of a more closely-integrated EC it seems probable that, in the long run, a revival of corporatism and a co-ordinated approach to wage–price fixation will be essential. At the moment this is not on the agenda of any political party and the abolition of the NEDC in June 1992 symbolised government attitudes in this area.

Controlling inflation means controlling prices, but most economists believe that attempts to do so directly are likely to be damaging and doomed to failure. The main emphasis, therefore, has been placed on limiting increases in pay, although this begs many questions about the causes of inflation, fairness between different interest groups and methods of control. Up to the late 1970s a series of incomes policies were introduced with varying degrees of success. In 1979 the first Thatcher government had no confidence in its ability to find a corporatist solution to the problem of pay restraint and this was an important factor in the decision to embark upon a monetarist experiment. The rigorous attempt to control money supply (M3) failed, but in the process heavy damage was done to British manufacturing capacity, and unemployment on an unprecedented post-war scale emerged. The lesson of the early 1980s appears to be that tight financial control is likely to be enormously damaging in social and economic terms unless it is accompanied by some other means of influencing wage–price determination in the private sector. The Major government has not learned this lesson and seems set to continue its reliance on heavy unemployment with policies which damage both British industry and the social fabric.

The essential alternative to unemployment and low growth is to seek new methods of pay bargaining which give workers reasonable assurances on both prices and comparability in return for pay restraint. This might involve national agreements on pay, prices and relativities in advance of individual pay settlements, together with measures for the enforcement of agreements. One important government input into such a system might be guarantees relating to levels of economic activity including employment. Quite clearly any corporatist approach along such lines would require a dramatic reversal of existing attitudes towards both trade unions and employer associations. In turn, those bodies would need to undertake changes in attitudes and organisation. At the present time such development seems unlikely and it appears inevitable that any significant increase in levels of economic activity will produce the familiar wage–price escalation and problems on external account leading to eventual deflation and rising unemployment once again. In the future, therefore, unemployment relief and related expenditure will absorb a high and increasing share of social expenditure and there will be continued pressures for cutting the Exchequer cost and promoting self-financing of other welfare items, in particular health and education. These tendencies will be enhanced if pledges to reduce taxation are honoured. Continued high unemployment will also exacerbate existing trends towards increasing social and economic inequalities with related consequences in terms of crime, violence, family break-up and a range of other problems (Forrester and Ward 1991).

Since the mid-1970s Britain has moved from a political consensus in which welfarism and full employment were regarded as fundamental, to an uncertain political climate in which these considerations take second place. All political parties have played a part in this transition. Behind the party political hypocrisy and manipulation lies a failure in economic and social analysis. In general, economics has either supported or failed to oppose the departure from full employment and the positive case for a full employment policy has received little support. Social theorists, while lamenting the adverse effects of unemployment, have underestimated the damage to welfare systems. Unemployment must now be seen as a long-term problem which will require important changes in attitudes. From the welfare point of view a return to full employment is highly desirable but the received wisdom in British politics is that economic necessities preclude this. The problem is not unique to Britain but the British situation is more extreme than most and as a result the social welfare outlook remains bleak. Continuation of heavy unemployment in Britain will mean the end of the welfare state as it was previously conceived.

Chapter 5

Social security
The cost of persistent poverty

Hartley Dean

The UK social security programme represents the largest single item of government expenditure, accounting in 1992–3 for 31 per cent of anticipated public expenditure (DSS 1992: 1), more than twice as much as is spent on either health or education. It is a programme which has grown inexorably in size, from 8 per cent of gross household income in 1965 to 12 per cent in 1990 (Piachaud 1990), and which the government projects will continue to grow at more than 3 per cent annually over the next few years (DSS 1992: 6).

At the same time, however, around one quarter of the British population is living 'in poverty', whether defined in terms of having incomes which are at or close to current means-tested benefit levels or which are below 60 per cent of the national average, adjusted for household size and composition (Oppenheim 1990). The proportion of people in poverty by equivalent relative definitions has approximately doubled in the last thirty years, in spite of the massive expansion of social security spending (Piachaud 1990). It is only if poverty is stringently defined with reference to below subsistence level incomes that poverty can be said not to have increased (George and Howards 1991: Table 2.1).

In the years since the 1942 Beveridge Report, of the five 'giants' which the post-war welfare state set out to slay (Want, Disease, Ignorance, Squalor, and Idleness) it is perhaps Want (or 'poverty') which has most changed its face. It is not only that the incidence of poverty has increased, but the causes and the character of poverty have changed as well and the very structure of the social security system is in many ways ill-fitted to the task of tackling this 'new poverty' (Donnison 1991a; Room *et al.* 1989). The 'old poor' whose needs were addressed by the Beveridge scheme were principally pensioners and families with children, for whom the risk of poverty was defined by the vicissitudes of the life cycle. The 'new poor' whose needs a modern social security system must also address are the unemployed, the low paid and lone parents, for whom the risk of poverty has arisen through economic and social change. This is not to say that the actual numbers of pensioners and especially children in poverty have not increased, but that, in recent years, an increasing proportion of the poorest section of the population is of working age (see Dean and Taylor-Gooby 1992: Ch. 1).

Since the 1970s, the proportion of expenditure going to people over pensionable age has therefore been declining (Barr and Coulter 1990: Table 7.2), but it still accounts for around one half of all benefits paid. What is more, the long-term trend to population ageing means that such spending will continue to make substantial demands, especially by the end of the first quarter of the next century when the number of workers per pensioner is forecast to fall from 2.7 to 2.0 (Ermisch 1990). At the same time, trends in family formation and dissolution since the 1970s have been associated with a doubling in the proportion of families with children to be headed by a lone parent (Brown 1990). There are currently in the UK over 1 million lone parents in receipt of means-tested benefits and the actual number of lone parents is forecast to rise from something over 1 million in the 1980s to around 2.8 million by 2005 (FPSC 1986). Benefits for the unemployed currently account for 11 per cent of benefits expenditure and, while this is less than in the mid-1980s, it is about twice the proportion spent in the mid-1970s (Barr and Coulter 1990: Table 7.2). Unemployment, which had remained at around 3 per cent for most of the 1950s and 1960s, rose during the 1970s and, apart from a brief fall below 9 per cent in 1989–90, has remained consistently above 11 per cent since 1981 (Dean and Taylor-Gooby 1992: Figure 3.2).

The pressures upon the social security system have thus been brought about by a complex combination of demographic, social and economic trends. This is the context within which this chapter will examine the social security policies of the three main political parties. Those policies will be evaluated for their likely effectiveness in tackling the 'new poverty' as well as for their implications in the expenditure–taxation–growth equation.

THE POLICY ALTERNATIVES

All parties have in the past shared a commitment to the social security system. None the less, in the 1960s and 1970s Labour governments made important reforms, attempting in particular to make more resources available for cash benefits and to reduce a developing reliance upon means-tests. In the 1980s, Conservative governments sought to devote fewer resources to cash benefits relative to GDP and, by deliberate reliance upon means-testing, to increase the 'targeting' of benefits. It has been argued, however, that the net impact of these policies involved 'less discontinuity . . . than is often supposed' (Barr and Coulter 1990: 333; see also Dean 1991). Meanwhile, the Liberal Democrats, although ostensibly a new political party, have declared themselves 'proud' of a heritage which encompasses such reforming Liberals as Lloyd George and Sir William Beveridge himself (SLD 1989a: 3). The parties have all been associated with the shaping of current social security arrangements and, in framing their policies for the future, may be regarded as having a common point of departure.

The Conservative Party

The Conservative Party has been in government since 1979. Its policies contain three components: first, established policies embodied in the various reforms introduced during the Thatcher years; second, recent commitments which are still in the process of being implemented; and third, the shift in emphasis or 'style' portended by the advent of John Major's premiership.

The principal Conservative reforms during the early 1980s were as follows:

1 From 1980, the government cut expenditure by changing the basis upon which most social security benefits and pensions are annually uprated so as to link them to price inflation, rather than to rises in earnings.
2 In the mid-1980s, new 'employer mandated' benefits – statutory sick pay (SSP) and statutory maternity pay (SMP) – were introduced, thus transferring the administration of most short-term sickness and maternity benefits from the national insurance scheme to employers.
3 Between 1979 and 1988 there were no fewer than 38 significant

changes affecting social security benefits for the unemployed (Atkinson and Micklewright 1988), most of which were intended to increase work incentives.

A second tranche of reforms resulted from the Fowler Reviews, set up in 1984 and culminating in the 1986 Social Security Act. The main provisions of that Act were implemented in 1988 and involved:

4 A significant shift towards the 'targeting' of benefits through means-testing and the recasting of the main means-tested benefits (through the creation of Income Support and Family Credit and changes to Housing Benefit).
5 The freezing of universal Child Benefit at its 1987 level and some reduction in the scope of certain National Insurance benefits.
6 The reduction in the value of future benefits under the State Earnings Related Pension Scheme (SERPS) and the promotion through subsidies of Personal Pension Plans and new occupational schemes.
7 The creation of the cash limited Social Fund which replaced the system of grants which had been available under the old Supplementary Benefit scheme and provides discretionary assistance with one-off items of expenditure for those on Income Support, usually in the form of loans.

In the 1990s, the Conservatives have set in train a further set of reforms:

8 From 1991, the administration of most social security benefits has been devolved to a semi-autonomous executive agency, the Benefits Agency (BA), and the administration of National Insurance contributions has been similarly transferred to the National Insurance Contributions Agency.
9 In 1992, the government replaced the current mobility and attendance allowances with a Disability Living Allowance and introduced a new Disability Working Allowance – a means-tested benefit for disabled workers.
10 In 1993, the government set up a further executive agency, the Child Support Agency, which administers new arrangements for enforcing child maintenance payments by absent parents.

Since John Major became Prime Minister in 1990, there has been a certain change in style of government and a new emphasis in ministerial pronouncements upon extending 'opportunities' to all citizens (Bennett 1991). However, as Alan Deacon has pointed out,

> It is important not to exaggerate the change which has occurred. The four central themes [of Conservative policy in the 1980s] – the acceptance of inequalities, the repudiation of government responsibility for unemployment, privatisation, and the restraint of public spending – all remain.
>
> (Deacon 1991: 20)

In 1991, it was announced that, after a four-year freeze, the indexation of Child Benefit would be resumed and provision was made for an extra £1 per week for the first or only child in a family. In their 1992 manifesto, the Conservatives gave a commitment to maintaining the value of Child Benefit (Conservative Party 1992: 21). Excepting this significant change, none of the central tenets of the policies outlined above has been renounced. On the contrary, the 1992 manifesto promised 'further encouragement' for the spread of personal pensions, although, in the light of recent pension fund scandals, it also pledged a review of the legal and regulative framework within which occupational schemes operate (1992: 8, 20). Prior to the 1992 General Election the then Secretary of State for Social Security resisted criticism of Conservative reform, arguing that they represented 'a significant advance for many families who really weren't doing at all well under the benefit system before' (Newton 1991: 7).

The one policy commitment clearly associated with John Major's premiership is the 'Citizen's Charter' (Prime Minister's Office 1991) which promises a BA customer charter, published efficiency targets and improved accessibility and quality of service.

The Labour Party

It has rather uncharitably been said of the Labour Party that 'whether or not Thatcherism has succeeded in reducing the public's expectations of redistribution by government action, it seems to have succeeded in reducing Labour's' (Bennett 1991: 98). Labour governments of the past have been concerned to devote more resources to social security, but the series of policy statements which Labour has recently published (1988; 1989; 1990 and 1991e) and its most recent manifesto (1992a) are characterised by considerable caution about the amount of resources which a future Labour government would commit to social security reform. Amidst the caution, however, are proposals which if implemented could transform the operation of the system.

The only immediate spending commitments are to restore the real value of Child Benefit to its 1987 level; to increase the basic state pension by £5 per week for single pensioners and £8 per week for couples; thereafter to maintain the value of Child Benefit 'at least in line with inflation' and to uprate pensions in line with earnings; and to convert all Social Fund loans back into grants, with a right of appeal. However, central to the 'opportunities for independence' which Labour would promote is a commitment to introduce a statutory minimum wage – initially at half median male earnings, rising to two-thirds over time. This is the most distinctive element of the Labour Party's programme, since it involves an approach to poverty prevention which is unequivocally interventionist and which departs from the principles of Beveridge.

The rest of Labour's programme consists of 'longer-term objectives' which would be realised 'as resources allow'. The most conceptually significant but tantalising proposal is for 'improved social insurance' which will 'reflect changing working patterns and expectations' (Labour Party 1991e: 40), and in which low-paid and part-time workers and the self-employed would be able to participate. The scheme envisaged is portrayed in terms of 'a new contract between the individual and society'. This would be a contract under which entitlement to benefits 'should not turn on a narrow contribution test but should be established by experience of the conditions which it covers – old age, unemployment or disability'; which would 'contribute to our goal of an independent benefit entitlement for women'; but which, in accepting that access to benefits should be universal, would be capable of responding to individual needs on a case-by-case basis (Labour Party 1989: 34–5). These are ambitious claims. A system which achieved such objectives would correct the most intractable defects of the Beveridge scheme, but the difficult detail of how this might be done is not spelt out.

Labour's longer-term plans also include:

1 A new National Pensions Plan, which would build on SERPS; a

'flexible decade of retirement' for all aged 60–70; new requirements on minimum pension levels payable by occupational and
personal pension providers; and the option of paying extra
contributions for extra benefits through the state scheme.

2 A new disability benefit with a universal component to meet the
extra costs associated with having a disability (however caused)
and a component to meet the income needs of those disabled
people who cannot work or can only work part-time.

3 A review of the needs of carers for the disabled and an
extension of the Invalid Care Allowance, which should in time
be increased at least to the level of the basic retirement pension.

4 Various proposals to improve means-tested assistance
(including the restoration of rights to benefit for 16- and
17-year-olds, a premium for the long-term unemployed and
disregards on child maintenance received by lone parents), but
subject to an emphasis that such benefits should be a 'safety net'
rather than the mainstream form of provision.

The Liberal Democrats

Of the main political parties, the Liberal Democrats are the most
explicit in asserting that the current social security system, based
originally on the concept of national insurance, 'has reached the
end of a noble life and is going to have to be replaced' (Ashdown
1990/1).

The Liberal Democrats are the first major political party to
advocate the idea of integrating the tax and benefits systems by
establishing a basic income scheme or 'Citizens' Income' (SLD
1989a and Liberal Democrats 1992). The concept which underlies
a basic income scheme is disarmingly simple, and if implemented
in its 'pure' form would allow the complex panoply of social
security benefits and tax allowances to be abolished. Instead, every
citizen would have a universal entitlement to a tax-free basic
income from the state, but would pay tax upon the whole of
his/her income from any other source. It is widely recognised,
however, that to achieve a basic income even approaching a level
sufficient for subsistence – say £60 per week per person – would
require a tax rate of around 70 per cent to finance it (see for
example Parker 1989). Since this is not regarded as politically
feasible, the Liberal Democrats, like most other advocates of basic
income or social dividend schemes, have contrived a complex

strategy for phasing in a partial basic income. The strategy has three stages.

In the first stage, the basic state retirement pension would be increased, reindexed and converted into a Citizens' Income for pensioners, but SERPS would be abolished; Child Benefit, which already functions as a partial basic income for children, would be increased and reindexed; the Social Fund would be reformed; and there would be various preparatory reforms to the tax system, with national insurance contributions and income tax being combined into a single broad income tax.

In the second stage, which would follow the first by about five years, a Citizens' Income set at £12.80 per week (but with a higher rate for lone parents) would be introduced for the rest of the adult population; Income Support, Family Credit and Unemployment Benefit would be abolished but, for those on low incomes, the Citizens' Income would be supplemented by a unified Low Income Benefit, which would be withdrawn (on a 70 per cent taper) as household/family income rises; Housing Benefit and mortgage tax-relief would be replaced by a single 'housing cost relief' (although existing recipients of mortgage tax-relief would have the option of retaining it); and the tax system would be further reformed and simplified.

In the third stage, the Citizens' Income would be gradually increased 'on a time scale dependent on the rate of growth of the economy'.

Provision for the sick and disabled would also be modified: the contributory principle for sickness and invalidity benefits would be abolished and all sick and disabled people would be entitled to benefit simply on the basis of incapacity for work; invalidity benefit would be increased by 15 per cent and mobility allowance would be improved (attendance allowance is not mentioned); invalid care allowance would be increased by 15 per cent and converted into a new Carer's Benefit.

Having decided to abolish SERPS, the Liberal Democrats clearly envisage a continuing role for occupational and personal pensions and they have plans to regulate occupational schemes and to require employees not covered by occupational schemes to set up a Personal Pension Plan. Like Labour, a flexible retirement age is proposed, allowing people to retire any time between the ages of 60 and 70, though they would receive a reduced state pension and would not be entitled to the full pension until they attained the 'reference' age of 70.

Summary

The above account has concentrated upon the main features rather than the detail of the policies of the main political parties in the UK, but the positions of the parties may be further summarised as follows. All the parties have come to recognise that the social security system inherited from Beveridge is ill-suited to present conditions, but all are now cautious about the amount of resources which can be committed to cash benefits. The Conservatives are attempting to retain the structure of the system as it has evolved, but continue to hang their hopes on 'targeting' for needy groups (through the efficient delivery of means-tested benefits) while encouraging better-off groups at least partially to 'opt out' from state provision. Labour seek to develop the existing system within the context of a higher wage economy through the introduction of a statutory minimum wage, to improve the level of benefits and to broaden the concept of social insurance. The Liberal Democrats seek to abandon the present structure and to move incrementally towards a Citizens' Income.

EVALUATING THE POLICY ALTERNATIVES

What are the implications of these various policies for sustaining minimum incomes, for the dividing line between public and private provision, for the balance between universalism and selectivity, and for the relationship between the state and the citizen?

Sustaining minimum incomes

Social security systems function to sustain incomes through the distribution of cash benefits. There is little agreement as to whether the object is to prevent or merely relieve poverty, or whether there is a definitive income standard or poverty line by which the success of social security systems may be measured. By themselves, none of the main parties' social security policies are likely to abolish poverty, but it is important to consider whether their stated objects are realistic, what levels of income they aim to achieve, how effective they would be in delivering benefits to those it is intended should receive them, and what wider consequences might follow from the distribution of incomes that is likely to result.

Conservative policy is the least explicitly egalitarian of the policies on offer. It is founded upon the assumption that the role of the state is to relieve poverty when it occurs, while relying upon the effects of market activity and entrepreneurial wealth creation 'trickling down' to raise the living standards of the poor. However, the evidence of the 1980s indicates that a rising tide simply cannot be relied upon to 'lift all boats' (see, for example, George and Wilding 1984; Walker and Walker 1987).

Labour's proposals are the most egalitarian on offer and contain the clearest commitment to the prevention of poverty. Even so, the caution with which the proposals are advanced raises questions about how much would be achieved in practice. There is often ambiguity in the pronouncements of Labour spokes-persons (Bennett 1991: 97). It should also be noted that Labour were responsible for introducing and intend to continue with the idea of earnings-related pensions, a feature which is not necessarily egalitarian: certainly, it can lift many out of poverty, but it can also contribute to the relative poverty of those with poor or non-existent earnings records.

At first blush, the Liberal Democrats' commitment to a Citizens' Income is highly egalitarian and preventive, but the problem with a partial basic income scheme of this nature is that it entails compromises which are fatal to the basic income ideal. The Liberal Democrats' scheme would, for an indefinite period, remain heavily dependent upon measures for poverty relief (the proposed Low Income Benefit) and progress beyond this point, even if it were politically feasible, would be entirely dependent upon substantial economic growth.

Turning to the question of benefit levels, the Conservatives remain committed to the greatest degree of restraint in benefit expenditure. Although the Conservatives lay claim to a growing level of real expenditure during their term of office, Townsend (1991) has estimated that, had the structure of the benefits system and uprating provisions remained undisturbed since 1979, a further £7–8 million would have been spent on benefits in 1989, and this in itself has demonstrably contributed to the proportion and distribution of people in households with below-average incomes (see SSSC 1991a). Both Labour and the Liberal

Democrats are committed to immediate increases in basic pensions and Child Benefit and to restoration of uprating provisions. The effect would be to raise the incomes and living standards of many of the poorest members of the population.

One of the key drawbacks to the Conservatives' emphasis on 'targeting' has been the problem of benefit 'take-up'. To the extent that 'targeting' has been made dependent upon means-testing, it has been ineffective. While universal benefits (like Child Benefit) and contributory benefits (like the national insurance retirement pension) are claimed by virtually everybody who is entitled to them, the take-up of means-tested benefits like Income Support (at around 80 per cent) and particularly Family Credit (at around 50 per cent) is far from complete (DSS 1991a: 22). The reasons why people on low income may fail to claim means-tested assistance are complex and intractable (Barr and Coulter 1990) and pose a major obstacle for any policy which relies on means-testing. Labour's proposals emphasise a shift away from means-testing in favour of what might be described as a 'rights based approach' (Alcock 1991 and see, more generally, George 1973; Lister 1990; George and Howards 1991). Labour's hope is that the new social insurance would provide benefits to which claimants would feel they have an automatic right. Similarly, the Liberal Democrats claim that Citizens' Income, because entitlement would be automatic, would present no take-up problems, though this is questionable because of the need to supplement Citizens' Income with means-tested provision. The Liberal Democrats say that take-up problems could be overcome through the integration of tax and benefit administration procedures (enabling tax liability and benefit entitlement to be assessed from a single return), but the practicability of such a system for delivering correctly computed weekly benefits – regularly and when needed – seems dubious.

The other critical question for any social security policy is whether it will create a 'poverty trap'. The term 'poverty trap' has several meanings, but is often used to describe the situation in which it is more difficult for poorer people than for richer people to improve their lot. As Hills has put it:

> Fundamentally, if the combined tax and benefit system *increases* the incomes of the poor and *reduces* those of the rich, there has to be slower growth of net than of gross incomes somewhere in

between. The 'poverty-trap' is simply the result of cramming all of this into one income range.

(Hills 1988: 32)

In another sense, a 'poverty trap' is a problem of incentives and arises when those who live on social security benefits are left with no incentive to work and to save. It is the Conservatives' preoccupation with the problem of incentives which leads them to limit benefit levels, especially for the unemployed. The Conservatives can justly claim by their 1988 reforms to have ameliorated the more perverse disincentives generated by the benefits system they inherited (under which a pay rise for some working families on benefits could actually result in a reduction in overall income), but they have done so at the cost of doubling to more than a million the number of working families for whom a pay rise can result in loss of benefits and additional tax amounting together to more than 70 pence in the pound (Parker 1989; Barr and Coulter 1990). The policies to which the Conservatives remain committed extend the poverty trap. Labour's approach, subject to the level to which the statutory minimum wage could be raised, does offer a possible solution. By raising the earnings of the lowest paid workers, the 'political ceiling' (Donnison 1991b: 150) of the benefits payable to those not in work could also be raised and would make room for the relaxation of the poverty trap. A Citizens' Income – if implemented as a 'pure' basic income scheme – would have potential for removing the poverty trap entirely by spreading the cost of provision progressively across the whole income range (although the impact on incentives to work and to save are hard to predict). In practice, the scheme proposed by the Liberal Democrats, throughout its indefinite transitional stage, would face the same poverty-trap constraints as the existing system.

The public/private divide

In a cash mediated market economy there are roles both for the market and the state in the provision of cash incomes. The provision of incomes, unlike the provision of health care or education, is concerned with the distribution of resources rather than with supplying a service or commodity. The considerations involved in deciding the mix between public and private provision can therefore be rather different (O'Higgins 1984). Nevertheless, pensions and benefits can be financed and/or administered in either the public sector, the private sector or both.

In the course of the 1980s the Conservatives in government have demonstrated that there are limits to which social security provision may be 'privatised'. Their attempts to entirely privatise the earnings-related element of retirement pensions (through the abolition of SERPS) were frustrated by the resistance of the private insurance industry. Attempts to privatise sickness and maternity benefits were substantially frustrated by the reluctance of employers to meet the cost. Even so, the government has succeeded in attracting 4.6 million people into Personal Pension Plans and many others into new occupational schemes, albeit at a cost of over £1.8 billion in incentives (DSS 1992: 16), over £5.9 billion in revenue foregone by the National Insurance Fund (NAO 1991) and a rise from £2.6 billion to £6.5 billion per annum in tax relief to private pension funds and their contributors (Parry 1991). The government also succeeded in privatising the administration of short-term sickness and maternity benefits through the introduction of fully state-funded SSP and SMP (although, since 1991, employers have been made to meet 20 per cent of the cost of SSP). However, the government retreated from a similar proposal to have Family Credit for low-paid workers administered by employers, partly because of objections that this would involve employers too much in the personal affairs of their employees. For the present, the Conservatives do not seem inclined to take new initiatives in the privatisation of social security, though clearly they do intend to allow a continuing haemorrhage of contributors from SERPS, and there remains scope for them to ease further responsibilities for occupational provision on to employers.

Labour clearly demonstrate the greatest commitment to the public sector, though they appear to show a far greater tolerance towards private provision than hitherto. Labour defend the national insurance system as 'the best deal available' (Labour Party 1991e: 40): 'The logic on which it is based is that together we can deliver greater security for everyone through social provision than anyone can secure for themselves alone through individual purchase' (Labour Party 1989: 34). In spite of this reasoned preference for collective provision, however, the Labour Party envisages the continuation of occupational and personal pension schemes, albeit subject to greater government regulation. The suggestion that social insurance contributors should have the option of paying higher contributions for higher benefits seems to anticipate competition between the private and the public sectors.

The Liberal Democrats are less squeamish about privatisation than even the Conservatives. First, their Citizens' Income scheme would require the wholesale abolition of SERPS and, not only would they encourage occupational and personal pension provision, they would compel employees not in occupational schemes to take out Personal Pension Plans (the feasibility of which for many low-paid workers must surely be doubtful). Like Labour, the Liberal Democrats would seek greater powers to regulate the standards of provision by private pension providers. Second, the Liberal Democrats' Low Income Benefit would be employer administered and paid to low-paid workers through their wage packets. The consequences of this for the distribution of income within the households of some wage earners could be disadvantageous (especially for women and children), and it would also provide scope for a considerable extension of employers' power (see Dean 1988/9).

Universalism versus selectivity

At the root of many of the differences of emphasis in social security policies is a question of principle: should cash benefits be paid to everybody regardless of financial circumstances (but ultimately recouped in taxes from those who do not need them), or should benefits be paid only to those who can demonstrate a shortage of income? Many of the issues already discussed – to do with 'take-up', the 'poverty trap', etc. – tend to revolve around the answer to this question.

The Conservatives, with their emphasis on 'targeting', are the most explicitly selectivist of the main parties and demonstrate a clear preference for means-tested or 'income-related' benefits over universal and contributory benefits. In 1988, their justification for freezing Child Benefit was that resources would be better directed through means-tested Family Credit. The decision to 'unfreeze' Child Benefit in 1991 would seem to indicate, if not a change of heart, a softening of the Conservatives' opposition to universal benefits in this particular case. Even so, Child Benefit has not been restored to its previous value and, while the precise direction of Conservative policy now seems less certain, it is unlikely that this recent move portends a wholesale policy reversal rather than a compromise born of a new pragmatism.

The main thrust of Labour's proposals is a return to greater universalism, not only through the restoration of Child Benefit, but through the extension of unconditional rights to benefit under their 'new' social insurance. While Labour are anxious to move away from the selectivity of means-testing, their conception of universalism is qualified by a long-standing Fabian tradition which encompasses notions of 'creative' or 'individualised' justice rather than strictly 'proportional' justice (Titmuss 1971), and which therefore countenances selectivity on the basis of need rather than income. This is evident, not only in the general rhetoric with which Labour espouses the cause of its new social insurance, but for example in its commitment to create a disability benefit which would compensate disabled people for the actual costs associated with their particular disability.

The Liberal Democrats' Citizens' Income represents in theory the universal benefit *par excellence*, though in practice universalist principles are subjected to some uncomfortable compromises. The abolition of the insurance principle in favour of partial basic incomes will result in less, not more universality, and the proposed Low Income Benefit seems likely to extend the selectivity of means-testing further than under any of the other parties' proposals. In particular, the proposal to abolish Unemployment Benefit (while tempered by the provision that, during the first year of unemployment, any earnings by a claimant's partner would be disregarded) would draw certain unemployed people into the means-test net for the first time since 1911. The problem is illustrative of the endemic contradictions with which Liberal Democrat transitional policies must contend.

The state and the citizen

The decade of the 1990s is to be one of Citizens' Charters, with all the main political parties publishing such documents (*Guardian*, 24 July 1991). While there are substantial differences in their conception of 'citizenship' and of the role of an 'enabling state', the common language of these charters revolves around greater choice for the citizen, greater efficiency in public services and better rights of redress for the aggrieved citizen.

In the 1980s, the Conservatives in government have espoused

'a partnership between the individual and the state – a [social security] system built on twin pillars' (DHSS 1985: paragraph 1.5). In the 1990s this conception has been elaborated by recasting the social security claimant as a 'customer'. When it comes to pension provision, ideas of the citizen as a 'partner' sharing in the planning of his/her eventual retirement, or as a 'customer' facing choices in the market-place, may have some superficial plausibility. But when it comes to provision for unemployment or lone parenthood, both ideas seem quite specious. There are circumstances in which people can exercise choices over how to distribute income in the course of their life cycles, and the Conservatives seek to offer a degree of choice between state, occupational and personal pension schemes. However, in view of the demographic and economic factors outlined earlier, the choices which people are obliged to confront can be extremely difficult: they may be akin, not to the informed choices of a high street shopper, but to the speculative choices of a high-risk market 'player'. The security of 'partnership' is eroded by a degree of risk for the 'customer'.

There are other circumstances in which citizens have no choice but to make a claim upon income redistributed from their fellow citizens through the agency of the state. The creation of the BA for that purpose does not create a customer–supplier relationship. It serves to distance policy makers from the responsibility of implementing distributive priorities which they have determined, the same purpose as was served in the 1930s by the creation of the Unemployment Assistance Board (see Lynes 1975). Although John Major's Citizen's Charter purports to make the BA accountable to claimants as 'customers', the BA's budget and performance targets are set by the Secretary of State and, even in the BA's first year of operation, its Chief Executive expressed fears that, without an increase in resources, performance would be prejudiced by the demands of rising unemployment (*Independent*, 26 June 1991). Additionally, the performance targets set by the government do not include targets for promoting the 'take-up' of benefits, although they do include targets for benefit savings from the detection, investigation and prosecution of fraudulent 'customers'. The effective delivery of benefits to those who are entitled to them therefore takes second place to the Conservatives' preoccupation with preventing benefits from reaching those who are not entitled (see Cook 1989). Citizens are viewed less as 'customers' entitled to a 'service' and more as subjects of administrative government.

In Labour Party publications the citizen is cast less often as a 'customer' and more often as a 'user' of public services. There is an emphasis on 'choice' for the users of public services as is exemplified in the proposal that contributors to the proposed National Pensions Plan would be able to opt to pay higher contributions for higher benefits. There is a general emphasis in Labour's policy statements upon promoting 'quality' in public services and upon the creation of mechanisms to allow users to complain or seek redress, but the only new form of recourse specifically envisaged for social security claimants would be a right of appeal against Social Fund decisions. In the field of social security, the state/citizen relationship is projected in abstract, almost Rousseauian terms, with social insurance being defined as 'a new contract between the individual and society' (Labour Party 1989) invited by implication to assume that the state, as the 'enabler' of this new contract, will be a benign or even neutral force. One of the weaknesses resulting from the lack of detail in Labour's 'new' social insurance proposal is that we cannot tell how this might be guaranteed.

The Liberal Democrats' Citizens' Income proposal, if it were to be implemented as a 'pure' basic income scheme, would radically redefine the relationship between the citizen and the state, offering the prospect of a new autonomy for the citizen and efficient, non-intrusive administration by the state (see Jordan 1985 and 1987). However, the high ideals of a 'pure' basic income scheme cannot be fulfilled in the compromised version offered by the Liberal Democrats. The extensive means-testing which would still be required, as is the case with the Conservatives' approach, would not be conducive to the personal autonomy which should flow from full citizenship. The administration of Low Income Benefit by employers would represent a particular violation of autonomy for low-paid workers. Similarly, the notion that some people would be compelled to take out Personal Pension Plans represents an infringement of free choice.

Summary

In the general climate of caution and pragmatism which pervades the current political agenda, there is a measure of convergence between the parties and a degree of tolerance by all parties towards principles espoused from different positions in the political spectrum.

Subject to this qualification, it is possible to characterise the Conservatives' approach to social security as the least egalitarian, as the one most disposed to private provision, as the most selectivist and as an approach which seeks to portray the citizen as a 'consumer' or 'customer' of state services. Labour's approach may similarly be characterised as the most egalitarian, as the one most disposed to public provision, as the most universalist and as an approach which seeks to portray the citizen as a member of a collective or community. The Liberal Democrats' approach cannot be characterised as an intermediate stance, but as a potentially contradictory one: it is a radical approach which 'does challenge us to answer fundamental questions about the nature of universality' (Bennett 1991: 99), but which in its pursuit of equity and the autonomy of the citizen could generate rather perverse effects.

CONCLUSION

This chapter has demonstrated that all the main parties have been responding to some degree to the consequences of economic, social and demographic trends. In fact, whichever political party or parties are in power, the policy choices to be faced are substantially influenced by external factors. In particular, the consequences of demographic change and the limitations of free markets cannot be evaded by government; the 'globalisation' of trends in economic functioning will increasingly force some matters outside the control of individual national governments; and social change generates demands and cultural expectations which governments cannot easily ignore or manipulate.

Population ageing and the pensions market

The Conservatives have sought to promote the use of private alternatives to state pension provision upon the grounds that the state will not be able to support the full costs of pension provision into the next century. Both of the other political parties foresee a greater role for the state than do the Conservatives, but they accept a continuing and (especially in the case of the Liberal

Democrats) a substantial role for a private pensions market. However, there are three issues from which none of the parties can escape.

First, personal and occupational schemes will not be immune to the consequences of demographic change since, as the 'baby boom' generations reach retirement in the next century, the resulting rush by funded pension schemes to realise assets may provoke a crisis in capital markets and so prejudice the returns upon pensioners' contributions (Ermisch 1990). Second, the spread of occupational and personal pensions is inevitably uneven and there is considerable variability in the extent and standards of provision by different schemes (Papadakis and Taylor-Gooby 1987). While a long-term growth of private pensions is already benefiting many pensioners, it also results in greater inequality in old age for a disadvantaged minority, since a free market in pensions cannot be relied upon to provide in retirement for those (especially women and the disabled) who have been on the periphery or outside the labour market. Third, as the Mirror Pensions Group scandal served to illustrate (SSSC 1992), private pension funds may be vulnerable as much to maladministration as to adverse market forces, and it is difficult to guarantee the probity and competence of fund managers in a large and expanding pensions industry.

The reality which any government must face is that it will have a continuing role to play in making adequate provision for those whom the private market fails or does not accommodate, and that it will have to adopt a proactive role in regulating the standards of provision in the private sector.

The UK in its global economic and political context

A central plank of Conservative economic policy has been to secure an advantage for the UK over its main competitors in the world economy by promoting a domestic trend towards an ever wider spread of earnings. However, a recent PSI report suggests that such a trend will present 'an increasingly insoluble dilemma' (Northcott 1991: 286). The relative fall in earnings at the bottom of the earnings distribution will compel the government either to set means-tested benefit levels so low that they inflict acute hardship, or else to allow benefits to rise above the lower earnings range so that people would lose all incentive to work or to save. It is likely that the UK must move away from a 'targeted' means-tested benefit strategy and revert to the use of universal benefits, rising with average earnings, 'in particular, child benefit, which can help cover the costs of bringing up children without at the same time reducing work incentives for their parents' (Northcott 1991: 286). This prophecy has already been partially fulfilled, since not only do Labour and the Liberal Democrats favour the reinstatement of child benefit to its previous value, but even the Conservatives have begun to make concessions in this direction.

The PSI report makes the point that this shift of emphasis would keep the UK 'more in line' with other EC countries such as France, Germany and Italy. This leads on to the possibility that the UK's membership of the EC will itself generate momentum for change in social policy which even the most reluctant politicians may be unable to resist. Although social policy objectives have played a subordinate role in the development of the EC and the EC has so far failed effectively to pursue the harmonisation of social security systems, the 1989 European Social Charter was intended to give new impetus to the development of social protection throughout the Community (see Ditch 1991). The directives to emerge in pursuance of the Social Charter have so far focused on measures in the employment sphere and have been intended to balance the economic and financial measures associated with the introduction of the single European market in 1992 (LPU 1990a, 1990b and 1991). Such measures have been fiercely resisted by the Conservative government but are favoured by Labour and the Liberal Democrats. The government, however – whatever its political persuasion – will have less opportunity to resist such initiatives in future and, towards 2000, we shall probably witness some measure of 'Europeanisation' in social policy, especially in the area of anti-poverty policy.

The UK's move in 1991 to 'opt out' of the Social Chapter of the Maastricht Treaty may ironically have served to accelerate the development of a social dimension to European integration, without necessarily ensuring that the UK will be excluded from the consequences (LPU 1992). This, almost certainly, will eventually involve some measure of 'levelling up' of minimum income provision, but it is unclear whether the benefits of this would flow, for example, to the unemployed and the low paid as the groups of greatest economic significance within the context of a single European market, or to children and the elderly whom public opinion throughout the EC regards as more 'deserving' (Room 1991). The emphasis of the EC Social Charter is upon the protection of 'workers', rather than 'citizens', and more pessimistic com- mentators fear this may assist rather than prevent 'the remorseless social polarisation and mass impoverishment which the single European market portends' (Townsend 1992: 21). Optimists and pessimists can agree, however, that '[t]he frame of reference is now clearly and firmly beyond the boundaries of the nation state' (Ditch 1991: 145).

Expectations of social security and citizenship

Future policy will also have to be shaped to local circumstances and personal preferences. For social policy to be effective it must work 'with the grain' of social attitudes and popular aspirations. Recent research has demonstrated that it is counter-productive to use social security policy as a means of halting or reversing economic and social trends – for example, by forcing social security claimants into low-paid jobs or into dependency upon family or relatives. Such attempts run contrary to popular sentiments and contradict the underlying value which people place on worth-while employment, on satisfying family relationships and on the availability of state support in time of need (Dean and Taylor-Gooby 1992). Social security policy must attempt to accommodate and not subvert the economic and social trends which shape people's prospects of employment and their expectations of their families, and it must function so as to reinforce rather than undermine people's commitment to citizenship.

Any social security system claiming to be orientated to the needs of the citizen must also be expected to give greater attention than at present to the demands of women and disabled citizens. Amongst the fundamental failings of the Beveridge scheme was that it afforded no rights of independent citizenship to married women or to persons excluded from the labour market through lifelong disability (Parker 1989). Although there have been incremental adjustments to the benefits system to take account of the changing expectations of women and the claims of disabled people, there has been no root and branch reform of the system's structure so as to secure equal citizenship for all.

So far as women and equal opportunities issues are concerned, such progress as the Conservatives have made in government during the 1980s has resulted largely from their being 'dragged along by the EC' (Baldwin-Edwards and Gough 1991: 157). When addressing the income needs of women, the Conservatives' 1992 manifesto confined itself to two specific statements: one commits the government to persist in encouraging and protecting part-time employment, upon the grounds that this is 'valued by so many women'; the other reiterates the recently formed intention to maintain the value of Child Benefit, upon the grounds that 'mothers should be treated equally by government, whether they work outside the home or not' (Conservative Party 1992: 21). In contrast, both Labour and the Liberal Democrats are committed to structural changes which would advance the independent entitlement of women. Labour's proposals for a national minimum wage and the structure of their new social insurance scheme are explicitly intended to benefit women, and such initiatives would be monitored by a proposed Ministry for Women. The Liberal Democrats' proposals for a Citizens' Income would establish the unconditional right to an independent income for all women, albeit at a minimal level.

It has been claimed that the Conservatives' social security reforms of the 1980s bore particularly harshly upon disabled people and their carers (see, for example, Oppenheim 1990: 74) and this is borne out by an appreciable rise in the risk of poverty which disabled people experienced in that period (see Dean and Taylor-Gooby 1992: Ch. 1). None the less, the Conservatives promise improvements to benefits for the disabled (see p. 92), although the changes they propose are less extensive and less structural in nature than those implied by either Labour's new social insurance or the Liberal Democrats' Citizens' Income.

While the political discourse of 'citizenship' in the early 1990s has clearly struck a chord in the minds of the electorate, the rights of the citizen to pensions and benefits must be accorded substance and value if a social security system is to retain legitimacy. The computerisation and associated managerial reforms undergone by the system in the late 1980s and early 1990s were intended to give effect to a 'whole person' approach to the social security claimant (DHSS 1982). Yet, in spite of the new significance given to the 'whole person' concept by the Citizen's Charter, according to welfare rights groups and civil service trade unions it has not yet been properly realised (SSSC 1991b). The DSS has taken 'a restricted view of what quality of service entails', and the highly bureaucratic approach adopted to managerial reform has been at the expense of more holistic and client-orientated alternatives (Adler and Sainsbury 1991). So long as the administration of benefits remains so bureaucratised and so tied to the control of individual behaviour, then benefit recipients (whether they be described as 'claimants' or 'customers') will not be constituted as citizens exercising rights, but as the subjects of administrative government. To the extent that they each claim a commitment to the citizen, this is an issue for all political parties.

All three parties seek to achieve sustainable economic growth, to moderate taxation and to promote an 'enabling' state. The differences between the parties are important, but to square the welfare circle we need also to look beyond the horizons of party political programmes. Social security involves the distribution of cash benefits in a manner which will protect the vulnerable from the risk of poverty. Risks may arise from trends which cannot be bucked, and the interests of those affected cannot be served by attempting to do so. The evolution of social security policy is a process which may be more or less radical but, in the present policy environment, there can be no single or definitive set of solutions. The direction of change towards 2000 will doubtless be affected by the mandate which the Conservatives won at the 1992 General Election, but the respective agendas of Labour and the Liberal Democrats have not been eclipsed, and the fundamental issues which this chapter has aimed to set out still stand to be resolved. On present evidence, expenditure on social security will continue to rise through the 1990s without reducing the extent of poverty in British society.

Chapter 6

Education
National success and individual opportunity

Peter Taylor-Gooby

Since 1979 the UK education system has been transformed. The long-standing trend to comprehensive schooling has been reversed, a new curriculum imposed throughout primary and secondary education, new examinations introduced, management restructured, further education taken out of local government and the most rapid expansion of higher education this century set in train. The issues of class, race and gender inequality have disappeared from the agenda, to be replaced by 'opportunity for all', 'the power to choose' and the contribution of education to 'national success' (Conservative Party 1992: 17). The Education Secretary of the 1992 Conservative government, John Patten, promises further reform: 'protesting teachers want ministers to go away, stop changing everything and leave them alone. But their expectation is absurd' (1992: 1). Both Labour and Liberal Democrats propose new patterns of curriculum and school management and changes in examinations and further education that are more far-reaching than anything envisaged by the Conservatives. Unlike the party of government, both opposition parties claim that education is in urgent need of extra resources. This chapter examines the forces that have promoted educational change, the policy proposals of the three parties and the factors that will influence future developments.

THE GOALS OF STATE EDUCATION

Education is not the first social service in advanced capitalist countries, but it is usually the first area of provision in which the state becomes involved on a mass scale to influence the experience of substantial groups in the population rather than minorities of the poor, feckless, mad, sick or disabled. The UK system was set up in the 1870s to plug the gaps in state-aided voluntary provision, at a time when government involvement in health care and social security was embryonic. When Booth wanted to gather reliable information on the lives of the London poor, the people he found of most use were not the poor law guardians, but the truant catchers employed by the school boards who brought 'the population . . . directly under schedule' (Booth 1902: 26). Even in the USA, the paradigm of liberal non-interventionism, a 'universal, tax-supported, free, compulsory, bureaucratically arranged' education system was in place by the 1880s (Katz 1971: 106). Education faces demands grounded in its supposed contribution to the economy and to the well-being of the social and political system, as well as the individual aspirations of citizens for self-development and opportunities for advance. Introducing the 1870 Act in which state education in the UK originated, Forster argued that both 'our industrial prosperity' and 'the safe working of our constitutional system' depended on mass schooling (Forster 1870: 104–5).

Economic, social and political factors have shaped the development of education ever since. Education is expected to provide an appropriately-trained labour force for industry, to socialise young people and to improve the prospects of voters. These themes emerged in the political agendas of all three major parties. All three set education a double goal in the opening sentences of the education sections of their 1992 manifestos: 'Conservatives believe that high standards in education and training are the key to personal opportunity and national success' (Conservative Party 1992: 17). 'Good education is the best investment for Britain's future. All girls and boys, from every background, must be able to discover their talents and fulfil their potential' (Labour Party 1992a: 17). 'British citizens are our greatest asset. Liberal Democrats will invest in people to enable every individual to fulfil their potential and in doing so build the nation's economic and social strength' (Liberal Democrats 1992: 31). The linking of individual opportunity and national investment is curiously similar between parties and curiously reminiscent of Forster.

The sentences quoted introduce discussion of rather different policies influenced by party ideologies. Conservative policy is concerned to widen individual opportunities by constructing an increasingly diverse system which offers the chance to compete for unequal levels of achievement, in keeping with a vision of an economy which 'rewards the industrious and thrifty . . . those who create prosperity should enjoy it, through lower taxes and more opportunity to build up personal wealth' (Conservative Party 1992: 6). Labour policies are designed to spread opportunities more widely through the expansion of nursery education and comprehensive schooling equally available to the whole age group, and through an attempt to make post-16 education for academic and non-academic students equal-status components of a new advanced certificate. This programme links to a vision of an economy in which 'no-one is left out of good training opportunities' and in which 'Britain's future [is] high skill, high wage and high tech' (Labour Party 1992a: 13). The Liberal Democrat programme takes the theme of equal opportunity further: 'our target is excellence for all'. Thus pre-schooling is 'guaranteed' for all who want it, all schools are to become comprehensive, inequalities in class sizes are to be reduced and a universal system of education for all 16- to 19-year-olds established. This programme is linked to a vision of the economy which puts the free market at the centre as 'the best guarantee of responsiveness to choice and change' (Liberal Democrats 1992: 6) and which sees education spending as 'essential investment in our country's future' (1992: 20). The problem of how unequal opportunities in the market are to relate to greater equality of outcome in education is not tackled. Both Labour and Liberal Democrats propose spending increases – £600 million over 22 months, and £2 billion a year respectively.

THE CONTEXT OF EDUCATION POLICY

Economic and social changes set the context in which party policies develop. The most important factor is undoubtedly the continued decline of the UK economy. This influences education in three ways. First, education is often blamed for economic failure on the grounds that it fails to train young people in the skills that are needed. An OECD report on the UK economy in 1991 referred to the 'chronic skill shortage and inadequate training of the labour force . . . the upgrading of particular and general training levels would appear essential' (OECD 1991: 78). The principal features of the UK system which emerge in cross-national comparisons are the greater resources given to academic achievers, and the low status of vocational training. In the UK the years of compulsory schooling are 5–16 years. Just under half of all children over the age of 3 receive some schooling, most of them 4-year-olds in primary schools (CSO 1991: Table 3.2). Some 65 per cent of 16- and 17-year-olds continue with some form of education, roughly half of them full-time in school sixth forms, a quarter full-time in further education colleges and a quarter half-time in the colleges (DES 1992a: Table 7). The full-time participation rate for this group is lower than in any major OECD country or any EC country (CSO 1991: Table 3.18), a fact which often leads to demands for the expansion of this sector of education, to enhance national competitiveness.

Second, economic decline cuts the resources that can be made available for state education. Over the decade from 1980, education spending fell from 5.4 to 4.6 per cent of GNP (CSO 1992a: Table 3.35). Conservatives are pledged 'to reduce the share of national income taken by the public sector' further (Conservative Party 1992: 6), whereas the opposition parties plan modest increases in spending.

Third, the assumption that education offers the key to economic recovery pushes the service up the political agenda. It was the only welfare state service to merit a separate section in all three manifestos in the 1992 campaign. It is likely that economic problems will continue, so that resources for educational improvements will be constrained at the same time as the political pressures for educational reform grow more intense.

The social factors bearing on education include change in the number of potential school children and students and changes in demand that affect participation outside the age-band of compulsory schooling. The demographic projections discussed in Chapter 3 do not suggest strong pressure on education. The number of primary and secondary school children will increase slightly in the early 1990s but will not reach the level of a decade earlier and will decline after 1995. The number of 16- to 19-year-olds will fall slightly from 3 million in 1990 to 2.7 million by the mid-1990s and will then return to the 3 million level by the end of the decade. These statistics indicate that numbers will be lower than the peaks of the early 1980s, so that the 1990s offer a favourable demographic climate for an increase in resources per head in compulsory schooling and an expansion of further and higher education.

The tightening link between educational qualifications and career opportunities and the pressure of rising unemployment, especially among young people, has fuelled the demand for education after the minimum school-leaving age. School sixth forms have grown by 32 per cent, college enrolment by 24 per cent and university enrolment by 29 per cent between 1980 and 1990 (CSO 1992a: Tables 3.16, 3.19 and 3.20; CSO 1984: Table 3.5).

Economic and social pressures bind education tightly to the economy, threaten the availability of resources and strengthen the demand for expansion. All political parties see education reform as essential to economic success. All promise to expand the system and to enhance individual opportunities. The policies of the Conservative government that has held power since 1979 dictate the immediate terms of debate in the 1990s. These are marked by a determination to constrain state spending, an emphasis on consumerism and antagonism to local government and to professional groups. Thus the five key issues in policy debate are: the link between education and the economy; the question of whether wider opportunities will lead to more unequal outcomes; the cost of schooling; consumerism and participation in education; and the role of local government and professionals. We consider these below.

Education and the economy: the new vocationalism

The subordination of education to the presumed needs of the economy involves two issues. First, government has to gain power over what is taught in schools, since curriculum, and the chief means of monitoring standards – examination and inspection – were in the hands of professionals who would not necessarily respond to the exhortations of politicians. Second, it has to decide how the needs of industry relate to the social and individual goals of education, and on this the parties did not agree. By the mid-1980s, all pupils took the GCSE examination, typically at age 16. The syllabus was laid down by Boards on which business was represented, but much of the assessment – up to 100 per cent in the case of English and some other subjects – was by course-work, and in the hands of teachers. For the academic minority, A levels based on the entrance requirements of universities were the principal examination, taken at age 18. Standards in schools were monitored by Her Majesty's Inspectorate, a highly professionalised arm of the Department of Education and Science.

Conservative policies for the curriculum are most far-reaching and most concerned to extend the power of central government over professionals. A ten-subject National Curriculum, designed to cover virtually the whole school syllabus between the ages of 5 and 16, has been imposed. The syllabus is laid down by centrally appointed committees under the surveillance of the Secretary of State. The curriculum does not apply to private schools nor to some experimental state schools. It includes Welsh in Welsh schools, but excludes non-European languages, effectively preventing much time being devoted to mother-tongue teaching for Asian minorities.

Schools are to hire their own inspectors, weakening the independence of evaluation. Teaching will be assessed through key stage tests administered to all children at the ages of 7, 11, 14 and 16. Tests in primary education are carried out by teachers, and in secondary education independent bodies are responsible. The tests are largely formal and depend on written answers to pre-set questions. The part played by course-work in assessment at GCSE was reduced to 40 per cent or less in 1992, and is likely to decline further as the examination is incorporated into National Curriculum testing. League tables of test results are to be published.

Both Labour and Liberal Democrat proposals are more flexible, offering five- and four-subject cores which will only operate from the age of 14 and will be supplemented by optional subjects. Both parties give technology a central place on the curriculum. Both parties will strengthen the power of independent inspectors, the former through an Education Standards Commission unconnected with the Department of Education and Science and directly answerable to Parliament, the latter through provision for more frequent inspections, conducted by the Department of Education and Science and extending to the private sector. Both parties will reinforce professional influence on secondary schooling through a return to GCSE in the original format. The system of key stage testing will be abandoned as will the uniform publication of results to parents. The Liberal Democrat proposals however allow for the publication of test results measuring the progress made by school students at the institution rather than the absolute level of achievement. This procedure eliminates the confusion of the standards of a school with the standards of the social group of pupils whom it attracts.

Schooling must serve the needs of society as well as industry. In this, Conservative policy pulls in two directions, the first concerned with the subordination of schooling to demands for a trained and graded work-force, the second with the preservation of social hierarchies. The 'new vocationalism' is evident in the central place given to technology as a foundation subject in the National Curriculum and the substantial funds devoted to developments such as the Technical and Vocational Education Initiative from 1982, the experimental City Technical Colleges from 1986 or the Technology Schools Initiative in the early 1990s.

The second approach is concerned with division and differentiation. The 1992 GCSE regulations make the examination more discriminating and provide for a greater range of possible grades. Some papers will only be open to a relatively small group of academic high achievers. After minimum school-leaving age at 16, the vocational emphasis is to be confined to those who are not academically successful. The proposals of the Higginson Committee in 1987 to broaden the A level examination and make it more accessible have been firmly rejected. A levels are to remain as the 'gold standard of post-16 education' (Clarke 1992). Like gold, they will be desired by many but held by few. However, a separate system of examinations, with a strong emphasis on vocational usefulness and on the development of skills rather than the assessment of intellectual abilities, was set up by the Business and Technical Education Council in 1983 and developed mainly in further education colleges, so that the division between academic and non-academic routes becomes clearer. School sixth forms, sixth-form colleges and further education colleges with their broader curriculums are to remain separate and in competition. The expansion of further education, like the expansion of higher education, is to take place with no extra resources.

The other parties propose to narrow the gap in status and in provision between academic and vocational schooling. Both wish to pursue a comprehensive system, leading to a GCSE examination which covers the whole of the age group. Both propose the integration of subsequent education up to age 19 for the Liberal Democrats and to 18 for Labour under unitary examinations councils. Labour propose the establishment of a broader five-subject A level in line with the Higginson Report. This will be integrated with the system of technical qualifications to lead to a common Advanced Certificate, that can be approached through a number of routes. Whether this will achieve parity of esteem is unclear, although it may be a step towards this goal. There will be a division between those in full-time education and others who will be offered a full-time traineeship for up to two years.

Liberal Democrat plans are more ambitious. They offer a massive expansion of educational provision, focused particularly on those over the minimum school-leaving age of 16. The overall objective is to raise standards and to break down the distinctions between academic and vocational education. The government departments of education and training will be unified. A single body – the National Qualifications Council – will co-ordinate a new course and examination structure for 14- to 19-year-olds which will cover both academic and vocational areas, and will also accredit courses of at least two days a week of training for those not in full-time education. Ultimately, A level will disappear as a separate examination.

There is a clear division between Conservative plans and those of the other parties. The Conservative plans retain the current vocational/academic distinction and apply it more vigorously to post-16 schooling. Both other parties wish to break down this division and generate a more flexible syllabus and examination system. It remains to be seen whether a division rooted in status differences that arise outside education can be healed by changes in education policy.

Opportunities, selectivity and inequality

A long-standing criticism of the UK school system has been its emphasis on differentiation rather than opportunity. The division between grammar and secondary modern education was ended for most of the country in the late 1960s and early 1970s, but numerous studies have shown that the schooling experience of many children is still divided on the lines of class, sex and ethnicity (Williams 1989: 182–3). Middle-class children are much more likely to receive extended education beyond the minimum school-leaving age than are working-class children, and to have more spent on their schooling – one study carried out in 1973 estimates over 40 per cent more (Le Grand 1982: 58). Boys are more likely to succeed in maths, physics and chemistry than girls, and more likely to attend university, whereas girls out-perform boys in English and humanities subjects (CSO 1992a: Tables 3.15 and 3.21). The move to comprehensive secondary schooling is not yet complete (some 10 per cent of children are still subject to selection) and occurred relatively late compared with most other European countries and the USA (Bellaby 1977). There is a small but powerful private sector, accounting for about 7 per cent of all pupils, but one-fifth of sixth formers and nearly half of Oxbridge entrants.

Selection has been criticised on the grounds that it restricts opportunities (Donnison 1970) and that it limits the full exploitation of the nation's pool of ability (Robbins 1963). It has been defended as preserving high standards (Cox and Dyson 1971), and as providing different educational routes for those of different aptitudes (Norwood 1943). These issues lead to problems in reconciling the various demands made on education in modern society. The needs of the economic system for an appropriately trained and graded work-force, suitable for an unequal labour market and the needs of society for individuals socialised to fit the various positions in a complex structure of class and gender inequality, may conflict with the desire for an extension of individual opportunity. The education programmes of the three main parties attempt to resolve this conflict in different ways.

The Conservative reforms of 1988 impose a curriculum which will fit the presumed basic needs of employers and allow for a variety of educational pathways designed to aid selection and to justify inequalities through individual success in gaining qualifications or entry to the more prestigious schools and colleges. Proposals in the 1992 manifesto, and subsequently in the 1992 White Paper *Choice and Diversity*, to increase the number of schools outside local government control and to allow them to test for admission, open the way to the reintroduction of selection at age 11 on a national basis (DfE 1992). The division between academic and vocational interests is to be preserved in the de-cision to retain A levels as set-piece examinations for a minority.

The Conservative Party has also indicated support for private schooling in the Assisted Places Scheme which provides a small number of bursaries (about 35,000) to enable children from low-income households to attend private schools. The means-test is administered by the schools themselves. There is no official research into the operation of the scheme, but independent studies indicate that the majority of the students aided come from middle-class backgrounds (Papadakis and Taylor-Gooby 1987: 96).

The emphasis on selection is reconciled with the demands for individual opportunity through consumer choice. Those who can afford it have the opportunity to choose private schooling. For the mass of the population there is the extension of choice through the loosening of restrictions on the numbers of students that schools can admit and the creation of a new tier of grant-maintained (GM) schools. Differences in resourcing and the selection of entrants may make it difficult for such a system to satisfy mass demands for enhanced opportunities.

Labour and Liberal Democrat programmes are both concerned to advance equality of opportunity: 'the rights of the individual must ... belong to all men and women ... those realities require that government provides ... education and training that fosters the ability of all young people and adults' (Labour Party 1992b: 7). 'We aim to create a first class education system for all, not just by providing adequate national funding but also through reforms which increase choice and opportunity for each citizen' (Liberal Democrats 1992: 31). Both parties propose to phase out the Assisted Places Scheme and to end the system whereby most private schools qualify for VAT and rate relief because they are classed as charities. Neither plans to abolish the private sector altogether. However, increased educational investment is justified on the grounds that it will aid economic development as well as enhance social equality.

Individual opportunity and the needs of industry are difficult to reconcile, since the jobs available may not match the aspirations of school-leavers. Labour's solution to this problem involves policies designed to curtail selection and to reduce the diversity of forms of schooling. Selection at age 11 will be ended. The Assisted Places Scheme will be phased out, and GM schools and City Technical Colleges brought into the local authority mainstream. The division between school sixth forms and further education colleges may be ended in a tertiary system, and the new Advanced Certificate may be approached through both academic and technical routes. Liberal proposals are broadly similar, the main difference being the lack of specific mention of the ending of selection and the greater emphasis on a broad curriculum open to larger numbers of 16–19-year-olds. Within this system of greater uniformity there will be wider diversity of possible curricular experience as central control is loosened, and stronger possibilities for transferring between different streams within schools and colleges. Thus the system emphasises choice within common institutions rather than selection by institutions and by consumers.

Labour and Liberal Democrat proposals raise three questions: first, to what extent will the system of opportunities in schools and colleges mask informal selection by professionals who guide students in particular directions, as opposed to the transparency of selection by institutions who either admit or refuse places? This problem is compounded by the second: both industry and society make demands on education in obvious ways. If education expands access to courses that have hitherto served as the passport to privileged positions, the outcome may not be wider opportunity but a devalued currency of accreditation. For example, shop assistants who were hired on the strength of school reports in the 1960s are now expected to have a GCSE pass in English. From this perspective it is unclear where the expansion of educational opportunity takes us in terms of individual satisfaction.

The third issue concerns the extent to which expanded access to education will release new skills for industry. While skill mismatches in some areas have damaged the performance of the UK economy, most commentators see economic malaise as rooted somewhere in a vicious circle of low productivity leading to relatively low rates of return which generate inadequate investment for modernisation so that the economy cannot compete in the most advanced industrial sectors, and is unable to afford high wages or support large-scale investment in the work-force which leads back to low productivity (Ball *et al.*1989: 33). It is difficult to see the extension of access to higher qualifications in itself reversing this process. The expansion of training may not enhance real opportunities for participants, and may not assist economic growth either, unless it is linked to programmes that will foster investment in the areas which people choose to pursue. Both Labour and Liberal Democrat policies highlight investment, but the pattern of investment is to be driven by industry itself in both cases. Labour's 'Decade of Investment' is based on enhanced investment allowances especially targeted at research and development. Employers are to be required to invest in training. Liberal Democrats reinforce a similar proposal with a statutory training levy of 2 per cent of payroll. Neither policy resolves the conflict between educational development, driven by individual aspirations, and training needs, driven by the requirements of industry. Individuals may find that enhanced further and higher education simply leads to devalued qualifications.

The proposals of all the main parties are dominated by concern about the fit between education and work. There is a clear contrast between the Conservative emphasis on selection in a differentiated system and the widening of opportunities in a uniform system favoured by the other two parties. However, neither approach appears free of problems: the selective policy may find it difficult to meet demands for greater equality of opportunity. The extension of access may collide with the requirements of the industrial system, if opportunities in employment do not expand at the same rate as opportunities in education.

The cost of schooling

Under the Conservative government participation in education after age 16 expanded, helped by a benign demographic climate with very little extra spending. The new constraints on local government spending imposed harsh restrictions on resources for schools. The real level of education spending remained roughly constant through the 1980s, only rising slightly as the costs of the expansion of higher and further education and of the reform of schooling became compelling. Thus Department of Education and Science spending stayed within 5 per cent of the 1979/80 level of £21.9 billion (in 1989/90 money, allowing for general inflation) up to 1990/1, when it rose to £25.4 billion. As the economy and the state sector grew, education declined in significance, from 5.4 to 4.6 per cent of GDP and from 14.5 to 14 per cent of the state sector (HM Treasury 1992: Tables 2.3 and 2.4).

Symptoms of strain have become increasingly evident. Pupil–teacher ratios, which had fallen from 23.2 to 1 in 1971 to 19 to 1 by 1981, only fell by a further 0.7 to 18.3 to 1 by 1990 (CSO 1992a: Table 3.34). Capital spending had fallen to less than a quarter of the level of the early 1970s by 1990 (Glennerster and Low 1990: 40; DES 1992a: Table 2.3). The Inspectorate reported at the end of the decade that nearly half of primary schools and 40 per cent of secondary schools were judged to have unsatisfactory accommodation (HM Senior Chief Inspector of Schools 1991: para 21).

Unless the UK economy expands more rapidly than it has in the past, resource constraint will continue. All political parties wish to double the numbers in universities by the year 2000, raising the participation rate for 18-year-olds from 19 to at least 30 per cent, and to expand further education. Labour and Liberal Democrats are in addition committed to an expansion in pre-schooling and higher spending on compulsory schooling. These policies raise serious questions about funding. The Conservatives propose to contain the cost of the expansion of higher education by substituting loans for grants, by continuing to drive up student–staff ratios and by cutting research in most institutions. There is no commitment for extra spending on further education. It is simply assumed that local management of schools will result in efficiency savings. Both Labour and Liberal Democrats plan to introduce new systems of grants for university students. Further education is to be expanded, most ambitiously by the Liberal Democrats, who offer at least two days a week to everyone up to age 19. Both parties propose to spend more on schools, to reduce class sizes and to make pre-schooling available to all 3- and 4-year-olds. Labour intend to commit a further £600 million in the first 22 months, with more as economic growth allows. The Liberal Democrats plan to inject the proceeds of a penny increase in Income Tax, estimated in the manifesto at £2 billion. In addition, the abolition of grant-maintained schools and City Technical Colleges would probably make small amounts available to the system as a whole.

It is impossible to judge whether the sums mentioned would support the reforms proposed. Total education spending in 1991/2 is projected at over £27 billion in current money. Labour are proposing a 2.2 per cent increase over 22 months, which would raise the annual budget from 4.6 to 4.7 per cent of GNP. The Liberal Democrat proposal at the most generous costing is an annual 7.4 per cent increase, which would raise spending to nearly 5 per cent of GNP. Before the spending constraints of the 1980s, education spending in the UK had remained above this level for nearly two decades. The changes that are proposed must be seen as modest. If growth does not return, they may be realistic.

Choice, participation and the consumer

The empowering of the consumer has been one of the main themes of social policy debate. The different political parties hold different views as to how this end should be achieved. In relation to education, the situation is complicated by the range of potential consumers for the service. Four groups may be identified: the students who actually receive the service, most of them young people; their parents and guardians, who in practice make many of the major decisions; employers who want a trained and graded work-force at the tax payer's expense; and society at large – the community – who finance education and have an interest in the socialisation of young people.

Almost all discussion disregards the first group. The interests of employers have received substantial attention as the links between school and work are drawn more tightly and the interests of parents move up the agenda as education becomes a political issue. The community at large receives lip-service. Mechanisms for consumer participation vary. The Conservative perspective models the parent/consumer as an individual whose interests are reflected through a quasi-market in resource allocation, while the employer/consumer influences curriculum, examination and school management directly. The Labour and Liberal Democrat approaches give more influence to professionals and to elected representatives by strengthening the role of local government in planning and administering the service. Consumers must work through consultation, lobbying and the ballot box.

Over the 1980s, the Conservative government downgraded the influence of professionals in curriculum, assessment and examination. Power moved in two directions: upwards to the centre, and to politicians rather than civil servants at the DES, and outwards to parents, employers and other service consumers. Consumer power was enhanced by two main changes. First, all schools and further education colleges must have a governing body, on which council nominees are in a minority and on which employers and, in the case of schools, parents serve. The governing body controls school management, staffing, salaries and other aspects of the operation of the school. Second, the power of local authorities to limit enrolment in popular schools was brought to an end. Schools were compelled to accept applicants up to the maximum number of places, and at least two-thirds of council budgets were to be allocated according to the numbers of students at schools.

The changes in effect introduce a voucher system restricted to the state sector. The local authority can no longer plan education in an area, because it cannot impose limits on admissions to a school or direct funds in a particular direction. Coupled with the publication of National Curriculum test results in league tables the result is the application of market forces to schools: the successful flourish and others decline, with the result that standards become more unequal. The operation of this market is facilitated by the publication of annual reports on schools and by the Citizen's Charter on education which is mainly concerned with parental rights to receive information and to appeal (DES 1992a: 16).

Consumer rights in education are further strengthened by the opportunity for schools to leave the local authority completely and seek grant-maintained status, dependent on central government finance. GM status may be sought by a school on the strength of a simple majority in a parental ballot, regardless of the numbers abstaining. A new governing body is formed with the power to perpetuate itself through co-option and the school's assets vested in it – while the obligation to pay outstanding loan interest on any improvements at the school remains with the council. GM schools are funded by central government at the same rate applicable to council schools plus an allowance for central costs, this amount to be deducted from the local authority budget. Thus councils are compelled to finance schools over which they have no control.

Central government capital allowances to GM schools have been generous, running at over four times the amount available to local authority schools (Taylor-Gooby and Lawson 1992: Ch. 8). By April 1992, only a small number of schools had pursued GM status – 134 out of just under 5,000 secondary schools, with 140 applications in the pipeline (DES 1992a: 12). Over half of these are located in low-spending Conservative authorities. The government plans to introduce further incentives to encourage schools to take this route, and anticipates that GM schooling will become the norm in the course of the 1990s (DfE 1992). It is unclear how this is to be achieved within budgetary constraints. The policy will either produce greater inequalities between council and GM schools in funding or will erode the financial privilege of the GM sector.

A further sector of centrally run schools, the City Technical

Colleges, modelled on US magnet school schemes, were set up from 1986 onwards. These schools were originally designed as demonstration projects, funded mainly by local business, but sponsors have been found for less than one-fifth of their funding and their long-term future is uncertain. Only sixteen such schools are currently planned.

Further education has been taken out of local control by the 1992 Higher and Further Education Act, which sets up new central funding councils to support these sectors on a national basis. Universities are funded through a complex system which includes both payments from the funding council payments for each student up to a set quota and additional fees paid through local authorities. The Higher Education Funding Council has driven down the unit cost in universities by insisting that institutions must take students additional to the quota, for whom they receive the local authority fee component only, in order to escape having their quota income cut in future years.

Consumerism has formed a central plank in Conservative policies designed to reconcile the demands on service users with available resources. Education authorities have become virtually irrelevant as school-planners and have no responsibility for college education. Conservative plans envisage the removal of many more schools from the local government sector. If this happens, the chief remaining power of the council, setting the local education budget, is unlikely to survive. Consumerism for schools is the consumerism of the market, operating within a rigorous centrally imposed framework supplied by the National Curriculum and key stage testing. Consumer interest is represented as effective demand, and those who are weakest receive no representation at all.

The other parties have rejected the notion of market consumerism in their discussion of participation in education. However, there is an uneasy balance between centralism, local government, professionals and the individual in both Labour and Liberal Democrat proposals. Both wish to retain some central intervention in the curriculum, to restore the position of professionals in relation to GCSE, and to broaden their role in relation to 16–18 qualifications and curriculum. The new tier of GM schools will be returned to the control of local government, as will the City Technical Colleges. The Labour plans come closest to a return to the previous system of local government planning and budgetary control. Schools 'will be free to manage their day-to-day budgets, with local education authorities being given a new strategic role' (Labour Party 1992c: 19). If the role of local government is to mean anything, it will have to include the power to close some schools, to expand others and to decide on specialisation within schools. If this is the case, the day-to-day budgetary powers of schools will be essentially trivial. Labour have had a long-standing commitment to the extension of comprehensive schooling on a national basis, which will reduce competition between different types of school for students.

An informal market has long existed whereby some schools are more popular, and are able to choose between applicants. Labour do not propose to bring this source of inequality to an end, for example by allocating places by lot. Independent enquiries will decide on school reorganisation, a system which will curb local authority powers to some extent. The consumer as student does not figure in the plans. The consumer as parent will have the right to participate in a home–school contract, and to complain to a national Education Standards Commission. The significance of these changes depends very much on the detail of the contracts and on the powers of the commission and the investigative resources available to it.

The Labour manifesto makes few commitments on further education. In opposition the party at first opposed the removal of colleges from local government in the 1992 Act, but later allowed the measure to be passed in the run-up to the election. Elsewhere, the party has advocated the amalgamation of sixth-form schooling and further education into tertiary colleges (comprehensives for 16- to 18-year-olds) which would facilitate the integration of A levels and vocational qualifications. However, this commitment is not included in the manifesto, nor in recent documents (Labour Party 1991c, 1991d, 1992b, 1992c). There is a repeated emphasis on the bringing together of the different aspects of post-16 education, but the integration is to be achieved through the unification of qualifications into the new 'Advanced Certificate' approached by a variety of routes, rather than the amalgamation of institutions.

The Liberal Democrat proposals also fail to clarify the precise balance between market forces and administration in education. The local authority will again have a strategic role which will include Colleges of Further Education. Council responsibilities will include guaranteeing a suitable place in education and training for every child up to the age of 19. This implies substantial powers for the authority in planning the local system. However, the ethos of local school budgeting is retained – indeed highlighted as a key point in the manifesto – and there are proposals to strengthen 'administrative capabilities' in the schools. Discussion papers indicate that local authorities will set budgets in annual negotiations with schools, and that teachers' pay will remain a central responsibility, administered through the school (Liberal Democrats 1990: 7–8). Open enrolment will be brought to an end. School governors retain few significant powers. In the discussion documents (and in local government) Liberals have been among the strongest advocates of comprehensive schooling (Liberal Democrats 1990: 4), yet this issue and the related issue of selection are not mentioned in the manifesto.

All three parties place great emphasis on responsiveness to the needs of consumers, yet there are contradictions in their positions. The Conservative Party has vigorously pursued a framework which strengthens the consumer powers of parents in a quasi-market, yet allows employers some influence, especially in further edu- cation, permits local authorities to set budgets and retains strong central control over the curriculum and over the support of the growing minority of GM schools. The consumer exerts influence solely as a market actor, and market freedom is limited by diversity of funding and by uniformity in the major determinants of school experience, curriculum and examinations – at least in the state sector – up to the age of 16. Consumers operate within a market where the product is similar but the level of funding differs. Beyond the age of 16 there is a clear divergence between A level and vocational pathways that is only partly driven by market forces. The influence of professionals and of local government is severely curtailed. The key question that emerges in relation to such a system is whether consumers choose schools or whether schools choose students: consumer sovereignty or selective schooling?

Both Labour and Liberal Democrats wish to allow teachers greater control over the curriculum, to reduce the role of selection, and to offer greater flexibility in switching between educational pathways. The emphasis is to be more on opportunity than on grading, and opportunities are to be enhanced by the expansion of the system beyond the age of 16. This approach stresses consumerism as choice within a system which is laid out by professionals who act to reduce the privileges traditionally enjoyed by academically successful people, those who stay on in school sixth forms and those who attend particular schools. Liberal Democrats wish to retain a role for local school management. The interests of schools may conflict with each other and with the plans of local authorities, for example over choice of pupils or over position within a school plan for the area. In such conflicts the local authority will have the whip hand. The central question raised by these reforms is whether expansion and professional guidance can reduce the difference in status of different educational pathways: consumer choice or hierarchy?

Local government and professionals

The differences between the party programmes emerge most clearly in relation to the organisation and planning of education. The Conservative emphasis on selection and on consumer competition in a framework set by an imposed National Curriculum leaves little room for local government or for professionals. One of the most far-reaching aspects of the 1988 Act was the introduction of a state sector voucher system (local financial management plus open enrolment) which destroyed local government planning. Schools expand or contract according to student demand, and any proposal for school closure or change of role can be defeated by opting out. Roughly half of the schools that chose the GM route were scheduled for closure in local authority plans. As more schools opt out, it is likely that central government will take a stronger role in deciding their level of funding. More recent legislation removes further education from the local government sector.

The power of professionals to influence the pattern of schooling is curtailed by stringent central control of the curriculum and by the new mechanisms for the articulation of consumer choice. The new diet of examinations substitutes central government power for professional authority in the secondary sector. More recently, government has directed attention to primary schools. In 1991 the Secretary of State set up a review of primary school teaching, to contribute to 'the radical rethinking now needed as to how best to teach children in our schools' (DES 1992b: 5). The report recommended that 'at the school level teachers will need to abandon the dogma of recent years' (DES

1992b: 54). It argued for a return to knowledge-based whole class teaching and was hostile to the child-centred approach endorsed by professional consensus (Plowden 1967). As the teacher becomes more clearly defined as routine delivery worker of a prescribed curriculum, her professional expertise is diminished.

The reduction of the curricular competence of professionals is matched by enhanced control of the profession through the creation of a new council for the accreditation of teacher training and the development of new routes into teaching for non-graduates as licensed teachers. It is currently proposed to sever the link between teacher training and higher education and base training mainly in schools.

The ambivalent attitude of Labour and Liberal Democrats to the role of local government in education is discussed above. Both wish to reintegrate GM schools into the local system, both are opposed to the doctrines of selectivity but both wish to retain some elements of local management in schools, Liberal Democrats more strongly than the Labour Party. This leaves the local authority in a strategic role, planning the overall pattern of provision in an area but unable to dictate the internal organisation of schools.

Both parties wish to see control over what is taught returned to professionals, with a dilution of the requirements of the National Curriculum, greater emphasis on teacher assessment in relation to GCSE and wider access to post-16 courses. Both propose the retention of teacher training within higher education and regard teaching as a graduate-only profession. However, both wish to set up accreditation bodies (coincidentally to be named the General Teaching Council in both cases) which will enable government to intervene in the setting of professional standards.

Policies in relation to local government and professionalism and education follow a pattern set by other policies. For consumer competition and selectivism to succeed within a framework dictated by central government, the influence of other agencies must be reduced, and this is what the Conservatives have done. Alternative policies that stress access and opportunity require a planned service (although planning does not have to be done locally), and are inclined to treat service providers as professionals who have the independence to protect consumer interests rather than as routine providers between whom the consumer chooses.

IMPACT: EDUCATION AND THE ECONOMY TOWARDS THE MILLENNIUM

The policy proposals of the three main parties fall into two distinct categories, each with its own agenda of goals and priorities and with its own pitfalls. The common theme that links them is the concern with the usefulness of education to the economy.

The Conservative agenda offers a system that is cheap to run and emphasises competition and selection. The organisational changes of the last decade have brought teachers and curriculum under the close control of central government. The resulting system allows schools to select pupils and offers basic schooling in different kinds of institutions up to the age of 16 and different routes to academic education or vocational training thereafter. There is no serious attempt to endow GM schools and council schools or sixth forms and colleges with parity of esteem. The university system is to expand, but loans will replace grants, so the students from lower-income backgrounds will suffer from constrained choices. This system will fill the labour needs of a highly differentiated economy effectively and cheaply, but will not meet the demand for equality of opportunity in an increasingly unequal society.

The agendas of the other main parties offer a different model of the goals of education and their relation to the economy. This model emphasises the provision of a common set of institutions through which individuals may pursue different pathways, but in which they have the maximum opportunity to gain access to a range of educational experiences. The idea of common schooling implies stronger state administrative arrangements to ensure that the most popular institutions are not able to impose their own conditions, such as selective entry or superior budgeting. The status of professionals is enhanced, although central government retains some power to intervene in curriculum and in the assessment of standards. The main problem lies in the question of whether the system will meet the needs of industry efficiently, or whether more individuals will achieve higher levels of qualification than the jobs available require, so that competition reasserts itself at a higher level. From the viewpoint of the national economy such extra education is simply wasted. In the context of the Single European Market it will be a concealed subsidy to our competitors, if they can absorb trained workers more effectively.

Assessment of the overall impact of the two models depends

partly on judgements about the kind of economic system for which education is preparing individuals and its relation to the state and partly on views on the social role of education. Here we consider two possible configurations of the political economy of the welfare state between which the future of the UK will lie (see Pfaller *et al*. 1991: 297).

The first is a high-technology economy resting on high investment, sophisticated government planning to provide the infrastructure and support that industry needs and a highly skilled and adaptable labour force. Such an economy is able to succeed if it can produce high-quality products tailored precisely to consumer demand. The second model is of a low-technology economy which competes directly on price in an open market. Since the second variant uses processes that are available world-wide, the cost of the local work-force in wages, education, training and welfare must be kept low. The UK contains examples of both high-tech and low-tech industry. It also has an expanding and divergent service sector in which labour requirements vary from banker to cleaner, systems analyst to shop assistant.

The model of education offered by Conservative policies fits an economy which is sliding towards the low technology direction, but which retains areas of high-tech industry. The overall cost of schooling must be kept low and many of the changes have swept away opposition to cuts. There is a strong emphasis on selection and on different routes to prepare workers for different sectors of the economy. Changes in the hierarchy of inequalities, which have generally widened the gap between better-off and poorer groups, and which derive from an economy with a large number of low-wage, low-skill jobs, fit neatly with selection mechanisms which enable the more privileged social groups to transmit that privilege to their children.

The alternative strategies of Labour and Liberal Democrats envisage different directions for the economy and different models of state intervention. More is spent on improving skills and abilities. Investment in education is linked to the creation of new and more sophisticated jobs as part of an ambitious overall strategy of economic regeneration. This programme is designed to shift the trajectory of economic development from competition on cost (which demands cheap workers) to a path where the educational level of the work-force can make a significant contribution to economic recovery.

Future education policy will be pursued in a particular economic, social and political climate which will dictate what is possible. The future as ever is uncertain. However, seven trends may be identified which are likely to continue whichever party is in power. First, the economic malaise of the UK will persist, with uncertain growth and with international recessions striking harder in this country than elsewhere. Education will remain high on the political agenda as an economic panacea, but resources for change will be limited. If, as some commentators imply (Bennington 1991), the UK is unable to compete in the single market with the high-investment, high-skill economies of the European core, the selective, limited-opportunity Conservative model may fit a bleak future better than the expansionary Labour and Liberal Democrat alternatives.

Second, demographic changes do not pose insuperable problems for education, but the increase in demand for further and higher education requires a response. Whether provision can be diluted so that these demands can be met without challenging economic constraints is essentially a political matter. Third, greater pressure on the system is likely to lead to a fall in standards. Competition will impose the reduction most significantly on lower status institutions, so that standards will become more unequal, unless strong measures are taken to prevent this happening. Fourth, inequalities of class and ethnicity will continue, though those of gender may decline during the 1990s – perhaps the only progressive change. Fifth, all parties are committed to some form of National Curriculum. Sixth, all are committed to giving consumers more information and a greater say in schooling. Finally, all wish to introduce systems of teacher appraisal, which will erode professional autonomy.

The future of education policy depends on issues that lie outside the eduction system. Education debate is inextricably linked to debate about the future of the UK economy, both as provider of resources and as the market which the products of the system must fit. Different parties offer different politico-economic visions, and the aptness of their educational policies will be decided by the success with which they are able to translate those visions into practice. Expansion and enhanced opportunity will only be viable if the political parties have the determination and good fortune to achieve the changes which will create the kind of society in which equal opportunity and high standards can become a reality for all in their working lives. Otherwise we have the second Confucian curse – not interesting times, but more of the same.

Chapter 7

Health services
Pressure, growth and conflict

Nick Manning

Expenditure on health care has risen steadily across the industrial world both over time and with growing affluence. However, it can be seen from Table 7.1 that the UK National Health Service has remained in the lower reaches of this area of public expenditure, measured both in terms of percentage of GDP and in terms of actual expenditure. Internationally, then, the National Health Service might consider itself one of the great successes of public finance efficiency.

However, this achievement of relatively efficient health care delivery has gone almost unnoticed, or at least it has been much undervalued. More often the service is castigated for its tatty appearance, bureaucratic insensitivity and uneconomic use of resources, and this image has enabled the most radical review and

Table 7.1 Expenditure on health care relative to GDP, selected OECD countries

Country	Total health expenditure,% GDP				GDP ($ per cap) 1987
	1975	1980	1985	1987	
Portugal	6.4	5.9	7.0	6.4	6,297
Greece	4.1	4.3	4.9	5.3	6,363
Ireland	7.7	8.5	8.0	7.4	7,541
Spain	5.1	5.9	6.0	6.0	8,681
UK	5.5	5.8	6.0	6.1	12,340
France	6.8	7.6	8.6	8.6	12,803
Germany	7.8	7.9	8.2	8.2	13,323
Denmark	6.5	6.8	6.2	6.0	13,329
Sweden	8.0	9.5	9.4	9.0	13,771
USA	8.4	9.2	10.6	11.2	18,338

Source: OECD 1990b

reconstitution of British health care to be successfully carried through by Margaret Thatcher before her political demise. The details of these changes are presented later.

DEMAND

Demographic factors

Health care is not consumed evenly over the typical life-span. Patients are disproportionately concentrated amongst the very young and, particularly, the very old. This pattern is common to all advanced industrial countries, where the very old account for something like six times the average per capita health care resource use (Robinson and Judge 1987: 7). Changes in the age structure of the population may thus have significant consequences for health care. Indeed, current projections (detailed in Chapter 3) suggest that the rapid future rise in the proportion of the population over 85 years old, which can be fairly accurately predicted, will ensure a rising burden of care over the next 50 years in all industrial countries. This burden has been mildly offset by a reduction in the birthrate, and hence a reduction in demand from the other major user group – the very young.

A further demographic effect arises from the relative spatial location of health services, and the population. There are two main axes here: north–south and urban–rural. The first is the health care aspect of the general 'north–south' divide (Smith 1989). Historically, the north has been under-provided, and hence has a claim in principle for greater expenditure in order to catch up with the south. This effect cannot easily be achieved by withdrawing resources from the south, and hence makes a net contribution to pressure for expansion.

The second spatial axis runs along the urban–rural continuum. Here, under-resourced populations can be found at both ends, in poor inner city primary care, and in remote rural areas far from major hospital provision (Morgan et al. 1985). While the former may be remedied by suitable general practice incentives, the latter raises a more difficult tension between the inefficiencies of small-scale provision such as the cottage hospital, and adequate access. Again, however, the pressure is towards a net increase in service delivery, to raise the level of care for both populations to acceptable levels.

Technological factors

Of perhaps greater importance than in any other social service, the effects of technological innovation have been highly significant for the growth in the demand for health care resources (Davis 1990). There are three main areas: diagnostics, surgery, and prescriptions. First is the expansion in diagnostic capability. A good example is the use of whole body ('CAT') scanners for the detection of tumours. These are expensive to purchase, maintain and staff.

Technological innovation in diagnosis is naturally pointless without effective treatment. A second area is thus to be found in the most glamorous and high-status area of medical intervention, surgery (and its associated intensive care requirements). Here we find concentrated some of the most powerful, and expensive, tools of health care.

Turning from the hospital sector, which accounts for some three-quarters of health care expenditure, to primary care, a third technological development has been inexorably driving up the pressure for increased spending, namely pharmaceutical treatment. This comes in two guises: the widespread expectation by both general practitioners and their patients that there should be a drug for every minor condition, regardless of cost; and the development of a new generation of expensive 'super drugs' for less widespread conditions (for instance, AZT for AIDS).

Clearly there should be great potential for technological developments to reduce demand through the efficient curing of some kinds of medical disorder. In general, however, the impact of technology in the foreseeable future is to increase demand, since it pushes people towards longer lives, and the age at which we know they will consume health care disproportionately. Only when technology makes for a healthy longevity, followed by a rapid and simple death, are we likely to see reductions in demand.

Social factors

Social factors affect health care demand in three distinct ways: the distribution of health and illness; access to and take-up of health care; and the very nature of health and illness itself.

The distribution of health and illness is not evenly spread over the population. Inequalities are ranged along dimensions of class, gender, age, ethnicity, employment, region, handicap, and so on (Morgan *et al.* 1985). To the extent that these are changing we would thus expect the demand for health care to change. We have already looked briefly at the effects of age, which are considerable. Another example is class (and for some writers, poverty in particular) which also has a major effect on the level of morbidity and mortality, leading to higher levels of need in lower social classes. This effect even carries over to the wives and children of working-class men, although for all these cases class effects tend to recede with advancing age (Morgan *et al.* 1985). However, to the extent that class differences, and poverty in particular, are growing (Silburn 1992), we can expect the demand for health care to rise. Ethnicity, unemployment, poverty or region are likely to be showing in large part the effects of class or, to put it another way, the evidence that there are significant non-class effects associated with these factors is thin.

Turning to the resource implications of access to and use of health care, evidence is strong in the case of region, class, age, gender, and race. For example, regional imbalances have been famously described by Tudor Hart (1971) as following an 'inverse care law', in which medical facilities appear to be distributed inversely in comparison with needs. Throughout the 1970s and 1980s there were attempts to deal with this through the resource allocation formula (RAWP) which required that increased resources were to be found for relatively under-provided areas (Morgan *et al.* 1985).

Significant class differences in health care use have been found to result from both the reticence of working-class patients in demanding health services, and the tendency for middle-class patients to 'hog' available consultation time, or to experience higher rates of referral for specialist care (Barbour 1989). Similar findings appear for ethnic minorities, with some very large additional differences in the diagnosis and treatment of psychiatric disorders. Again, the elimination of these inequalities implies an expansion in resource provision.

This last point leads to the third area in which social factors have resource implications, the question of what exactly health and illness are. Class differences have been identified, for example, where working-class patients expect their bodies to 'wear out' with age, and expectations of reasonably good health decline amongst the very old (Barbour 1989). A health-threatening lifestyle and diet, which show marked class variation, have also been highlighted in recent policy documents concerned with prevention (discussed on p. 149). Clearly to the extent that a middle-class *Weltanschauung* spreads, and patients' and doctors' expectations rise, demand for health care will increase. Developments such as the Patient's Charter can only be expected to encourage this.

However, there may be countervailing resource implications of changes in health 'beliefs'. For example, high rates of hospitalisation and technological intervention for childbirth have come about in response to professional interests, not women's health needs, and this may even have resulted in a net damage to women's health. This could be an area for the saving of resources.

Political factors

We can organise our discussion of this source of demands for health care resources into 'micro' and 'macro' politics. By the first is meant simply the internal life of the health service – the distribution of and struggles for power in the everyday life of the hospital, and community health facility. By the second is meant the more formal political processes of government, administration, and trade union and professional organisation.

Micro-political factors with a bearing on resource use have traditionally centred around the awesome power of the consultants, and their jealous possession of clinical autonomy. For many years after the setting up of the National Health Service, doctors were able to make clinical decisions without regard to the costs involved, which led to a steady rise in demand for resources. However, this did not go unremarked, and even as early as 1956, with the deliberations of the Guillebaud Committee, it was noted that Bevan's original expectation that a truly National Health Service would ultimately lead to a reduction in expenditure as the 'pool' of sickness was eliminated, was unrealistic.

Turning towards macro-political factors, pressure towards the more careful planning of health care developed from the early 1960s, for example in Enoch Powell's famous target aimed at the complete elimination of mental hospitals. Until the late 1980s, attempts by government to exercise greater control over the NHS were manifested in repeated reorganisations of its internal structure, with the imposition of a classic bureaucratic form of hierarchical links of accountability upwards, and delegation downwards (Levitt and Wall 1984). This was imposed more successfully over the salaried staff within the hospital services, through the progressive tightening of budgets (for instance the RAWP formula to rectify geographical inequalities), than within general practice, where a traditional contractual arrangement gave doctors the clinical freedom of independent practitioners. However, it made only limited inroads into the autonomy of doctors and the principle of clinical freedom to determine where resources went, and which needs were to have priority. Since the late 1980s, a radical new assault on the power of the medical profession has taken place, this time with more success. The government has reorganised both the hospital and community services into an open contract-based system in which they closely control District Health Authorities as purchasers of health care from a variety of state, private and voluntary providers.

Political factors have therefore worked in contradictory directions: expansionary at the micro level, but restrictive at the macro level. Recently the latter has been getting the upper hand, and the NHS is now under closer political control than it has ever been. However, the room for efficiency savings thereby sought must be limited, given the historically low cost of the NHS we noted at the beginning of the chapter; more likely will be the greater ability of governments to shape the development and focus of health care, where they judge that clinical freedom is not being exercised in a desired direction. Clearly, political factors can limit and have limited demand, in the sense that the culture of the NHS both at the micro- and macro-political levels has been for a 'no frills' service where only serious medical problems will be dealt with. Indeed, this is one of the factors that observers from other countries remark upon to explain the relatively low cost of the NHS by international standards (Meyer 1990). It is even more notable, given that the historically low cost to consumers at the point of consumption should, according to micro-economic ortho-doxy, lead to relatively high levels of demand for a 'free' good.

Economic factors

It might be thought at first glance that the main economic factor related to the demand for and supply of health care resources would be the level of affluence of a country. The figures presented earlier in Table 7.1 suggest that there is some truth in this, and hence future economic growth can be expected to generate demands for relatively more health care. However, as is also apparent in Table 7.1, there is a wide variation in the proportion of GNP that countries devote to health care. Given the clinical ignorance of consumers and the professional power of doctors, this is as much a case of supply generating demand through medical innovation and political control as it is simply that consumers in some countries want more. Indeed, it would be reasonable to suggest that the comparatively low level of health care expenditure in the UK, in the face of an effective zero price to the consumer at the point of consumption, must give rise to chronic unfulfilled demand. This is the major economic factor placing demand pressure on any UK government, and one that was expressed by both the profession and the public with particular acrimony in the later years of the Thatcher administration (Taylor-Gooby 1987).

Within this overall situation there are a number of other economic factors which affect demand. One is the 'relative price effect' of the high labour costs of health care, where both the unsubstitutability of labour for machines, and the ability of professions and unionised public sector workers to bid up their wages, make costs difficult to contain. Moreover, technical innovation, which might for example reduce labour costs in a manufacturing plant, typically leads to service expansion in health care either directly by creating new needs out of yesterday's research, or by stimulating 'knock-on' developments such as new surgical or pharmaceutical requirements.

There are other factors, however, which might ease the demand pressure. These have been summed up in the twin health policy mantras of 'effectiveness' and 'efficiency' (Cochrane 1972). The first refers to the fact that some medical procedures do not actually produce the beneficial outcomes that are intended, for example the use of the major tranquillizers for psychiatric patients, or transplant surgery. The second is related to inefficient health practices which, while effective, are not necessary, such as the length of time patients spend in a hospital bed for post-operative recovery. Unfortunately, with the ageing of the population and the growing importance of chronic health disorders, 'efficiency' and 'effectiveness' savings that could be made in the past will be more difficult to find in the future.

A final set of economic factors of relevance here concerns the interface between the public and private economies. We can divide them simply into the production and consumption of health care goods. Much of the technical, pharmaceutical, and physical material used in the NHS is produced in the private sector. While in some areas it has been argued that the NHS has the advantage of a virtual monopsony, for example over medical pay, in others it is seen as the victim of production monopolies which allow suppliers to extract excess profits. British Oxygen, and some of the bigger pharmaceutical companies with patents over new drugs, have been criticised for raising prices, and hence health care costs (Klass 1975). The latter also employ a battery of sales staff to persuade doctors to use their methods of treatment.

As far as the private market for health care is concerned, many observers would see it as making available new resources for health care in response to the excess demand identified earlier as a feature of the UK situation. In fact at present it funds a relatively small and very discrete part of health care activity (for example elective minor surgery), such that it provides little extra for the major functional demands made on the NHS. However, it may in the future make a bigger contribution to the provision of the growing incidence of chronic ill health as the population ages, and where there is a much less clear role for health care intervention as opposed to community care. In this respect, some of the anticipated future demand arising from demographic changes may be met from the private sector.

PARTY POLICY PROPOSALS

The first part of this chapter has identified a complex set of factors which affect demand for health care, usually in an upward direction. In this part, we will review the policies that have either been proposed or adopted by the different parties in recent years. Since this has been an era dominated by the Conservative Party, the review will be structured around government policy as it has evolved, with alternatives proposed by the other parties noted as appropriate.

Bevan's expectation of a reduction in health care activity as the general health of the population improved was wrong. Although the Guillebaud Committee was set up in 1953 to examine the continued growth of expenditure, little action was taken until the 1974 reorganisation introduced the 'managerial' era of the NHS

Table 7.2 UK expenditure on the NHS, selected years 1982–91

	1982–3	1984–5	1986–7	1988–9	1990–1
Total £ billion	11,478	13,050	14,808	18,181	21,570
Cash increase (%)	9.4	7.2	7.5	11.2	10.7
Inflation (%)	7.4	6.0	6.3	10.0	6.9
Real increase (%)	1.9	1.2	1.2	1.1	3.6

Source: Day and Klein 1991: 42

which has gathered momentum ever since. The 1974–9 period of Labour office, while it saw some keen debate, for example over pay-beds, did not challenge the new managerialism, since the fault line continued to be between the state and the medical profession rather than within the state. The Labour Party needed the new structure just as much as its rivals as a means of increasing its control over the NHS.

After 1979 the desire to change the NHS built up slowly within the Conservative government. Initially the Thatcher government was preoccupied with economic policy, and subsequently the Falklands War. Social expenditure was marked by cuts in housing, and severe restraints in education and social security, but the NHS escaped relatively unscathed, attention still being focused on administrative structures which were further modified in 1982. During the second term however, the financial squeeze began, as is evident from Table 7.2.

Historically, a 2 per cent annual rise has been expected in inflation-adjusted revenue for the NHS to offset the effects of high labour costs, and demographic effects on needs (Robinson and Judge 1987). Rises below this level represent a real cut in resources, and a reduction in service in relation to needs. From 1984 up to 1990, such a squeeze took place, until the two years of relative expansion following the radical 1989 reform proposals and leading up to the 1992 election. It was pronounced that the shortfall could be made up through efficiency savings made possible by the new injection of private sector managerial expertise set out in the 1983 Griffiths Report; and to a certain extent this was achieved, as lengths of hospital stays were cut, costs per acute case fell, and the number of hospital patients treated rose (Day and Klein 1991).

However, the medical profession was very unhappy with this continuing pressure to make up revenue shortages through efficiency savings, and late in 1987 a joint statement by the presidents of the Royal Colleges warned that the NHS faced ruin. Mrs Thatcher was furious, and quickly set up a review, noted both for her own involvement and the absence of representatives of the medical establishment.

The 1991 NHS reforms

The main thrust of Mrs Thatcher's proposals rested directly on the ideas of Alain Enthoven. He argued that the problems in the NHS included the following (Enthoven 1991: 61–4). It was inflexible, with the government unwilling to increase expend-iture, consultants and general practitioners on contracts which protected their autonomy, and a relatively unionised labour force. There was no serious incentive for efficiency – nothing would happen to a hospital with above average costs: indeed, it might well be 'rewarded' with fewer referrals if its queues were growing. Centrally determined working conditions prevented local flexibility to deal with local pressures and opportunities. The ethos of the service was provider-dominated, with little incentive to meet patients' needs or wants: for example, the use of a queue rather than a realistic appointment system for surgical patients. Finally there was insufficient accountability for the costs and quality of the output of the service, which was (in a slightly mystical way) seen to be impossible to define clearly, and for which there was very poor management information on items such as the costs and quality of particular cases.

The solution was the internal market. The main innovation here was to separate the purchasing of health care from its provision. The District Health Authority would receive needs-adjusted per capita payments from the government, unconnected with the provision of services, thus incidentally making redundant the old RAWP formula for eradicating inter-regional inequalities. Hospitals and general practitioners would sell their services to the District Health Authority, but without their traditional monopoly of supply. As an encouragement to further independence of provision, the 1989 White Paper introduced the possibility of hospitals becoming self-governing trusts, and large general practices becoming independent budget holders. Consultants would be hired and rewarded locally, in a financial system designed for much greater local autonomy (DoH 1989).

This system was introduced in 1991, and in the run up to the 1992 election it was naturally subject to very close scrutiny by parties opposed to the government, as well as by government spokespeople concerned to demonstrate its virtues. Since health care is arguably the primary domestic social policy battleground, it comes as no surprise to note, as we did in Table 7.2, that the government increased NHS spending very markedly in the year before and after the introduction of the new system. It is not expected that with a fourth term safely in the bag, and the continuing problems of the recession, the government will maintain this high level of resource expansion in the NHS.

A further innovation has been the health element of Major's Citizen's Charter initiative. This, the Patient's Charter (DoH 1992), is designed to reassure the public about quality in the health service. The Charter, which came into effect on 1 April 1992, does three things: in addition to confirming existing rights (for example to health care on the basis of need), it offers three new guaranteed rights – a maximum of two years' wait for admission, prompt investigation of complaints, and details of local services – including local and national 'charter standards'. Second and third, it spells out these local and national charter rights which offer a range of targets concerned with issues of quality, such as other types of waiting times, and staff respect for patients.

Party criticisms

Many criticisms of the reforms can be usefully examined through the proposals of the other parties. As in so many areas these have tended to be dominated by the government's proposals, which have successfully set the terms of political debate. We can examine these through a number of themes.

Funding

The first is in the area of funding, and the possibility of non-state funding of health care. The Labour Party's view is that the NHS reforms constitute a 'three-fold threat': underfunding, commercialisation, and privatisation (Harman 1992). This has resulted in the closure of hospitals and hospital beds, the growth of waiting lists, the encouragement of private health care through tax relief on insurance, and the use of private facilities by District

Health Authorities. The Labour Party is concerned about the growth of non-state funding because it will encourage a growth in inequalities of access between rich and poor, and the possibility of a two-tier health service.

Labour's alternative is to redress underfunding through the increase of funds to the NHS by £3 billion per annum, and to reverse the internal market and hospital trust status which it believes are the main encouragement to commercial and private practice medicine within the NHS. As the Labour Party Shadow Health Secretary argued:

> You cannot build a hi-tech modern health service on the foundations of the raffle, the car boot sale and the flag day. It is no use having a tax cut if the casualty department is closed when you need it. It is no use having a tax cut if your operation is cancelled because they closed the beds to pay for it. That is why we will use the tax dividend from growth not to cut taxes, but to heal the cuts in our public services. That is why we will seek over the lifetime of a Labour Parliament to restore the underfunding of the past decade in the NHS.
>
> (Cook 1991b)

Instead, a system of 'activity based' budgeting would repay health authorities for actual work done, and include incentives for increasing workloads – hence also tackling the perverse incentives in the old arrangements criticised earlier by Enthoven. There has been some ambivalence as to whether any vestige of the purchaser–provider split should be maintained, since in 1990 Labour initially included a rather similar distinction, between strategic (health planning) and operational (running services) boards within District Health Authorities. In the run up to the general election – perhaps in order to emphasise policy differences – this idea was quietly dropped.

The opportunities for private–public integration which the Labour Party fears are to be firmly discouraged by withdrawing tax incentives, banning full-time consultants from private practice during normal hours, and closer regulation. This is a matter of some urgency for Labour, as such integration is developing rapidly – for example, non-trust hospitals are now using spare capacity, caused by lower rates of District Health Authority purchase, to offer private surgery in NHS wards (*Sunday Times*, 25 May 1992: 1).

The Liberal Democrats also consider that many of the problems in the NHS result from underfunding, and at the 1987 election took pride in the fact that they were prepared to make greater funding commitments to the NHS than were the Labour Party. They suggested a minimum of 2 per cent real increase per year to cover the demographic and technological effects we have already discussed, plus a number of earmarked commitments: more money into the old RAWP mechanism to iron out regional imbalances; more capital spending; better pay; better resourced primary health care 'teams'; better screening, and so on. Their case, set out in *Prescription for Health* (SLD 1989c), begins from the observation that internationally, Britain spends relatively little on health care, and they argue therefore that this is not a problem of economic capacity but of political commitment. They are moreover firmly opposed to state subsidies to the private sector in the form of tax relief on health insurance, since they argue that the private sector does not relieve demand on the NHS. Like the Labour Party, they are publicly opposed to a two-tier service which they believe the current government is creating. Nevertheless, they are prepared to tolerate the private sector, but clearly wish to favour charities and non-profit agencies first, with tougher controls over potential 'rogue' practitioners.

While not opposed to competitive tendering and contracting out (they have no loyalties to public sector trade unions in this respect), the Liberal Democrats are also unhappy with the idea of hospital trusts and GP fund-holding. They frequently use the experience of the USA to argue that mixed hospital ownership, and the emulation by GPs of 'health maintenance organisations', will merely lead to greater regional inequalities and greater administrative costs, and in the end will restrict patient choice through expenditure constraint; they argue that the limited internal market that already existed provided greater patient choice than will the new mechanism.

In their 1992 manifesto the Liberal Democrats made clear that they wished to abolish the internal market, GP fund-holding, and the independence of hospital trusts. While in 1989 they examined seriously the Swedish option of a local government take-over of the NHS, by 1992 they fell back on a common structure of 'local management of hospitals and community units', separate from but parallel to local government.

Quality

A second theme concerns the quality of health care, and the rights of patients. Labour policy is to redress some of the weaknesses of the 'old' NHS through a Health Quality Commission, a Health Technology Commission and a Charter for Patients (Cook 1990). The commissions are designed to set national standards for services and health technology, to monitor and evaluate, and foster innovation of both services and their monitoring through patient experiences and treatment outcomes. The Charter provides for nineteen rights (twenty by 1992 – Labour Party 1992a). Many, like Major's Charter, already exist; most of the others concern a similar range of quality issues, while none has the potential resource implications of the guarantee of a waiting list time-limit.

The Liberal Democrats (1989) claim to have been the first to suggest the idea of a charter, now common to all parties, to guarantee certain rights to public services of a definite standard. Their outline contains much the same as the government's, including an as yet unspecified commitment to limited waiting times. Otherwise their route to quality is through higher funding, a unified service, and local management links with local communities.

Prevention

A third theme is about the general direction in which the Health Service is moving, in particular the relative balance between curing ill health and the promotion of good health. In addition to his charter initiative, John Major also took soundings from health experts in the spring of 1991 about the future direction for health care, and a Green Paper subsequently appeared in June 1991 entitled *The Health of the Nation*. (At the same time the Labour Party tried to upstage this with a discussion paper entitled *The Better Way to a Healthy Britain* (Cook 1991a).) The government admits that the scope for prevention of ill health arises from some of the processes highlighted earlier in this chapter: Britain's health levels compare poorly with international achievements; there are significant variations in health by class, race, and region; there are also significant variations in the quantity and quality of health care provision. They argue that the constraints to improvement are those of knowledge and resources, and suggest that key areas should be selected on the basis that they are substantially harmful in terms of both morbidity and mortality, have good scope for improvement, and for which specific targets can be set. For example, on this basis heart disease would be in, but cancer would not (DoH 1991b).

In response to this analysis (which is actually quite well rehearsed in non-government circles – Williams *et al*. 1991), there is an interesting divergence in response. The government is almost exclusively concerned with target setting, for example a 30 per cent reduction in coronary heart disease and stroke mortality below the age of 65 by the year 2000, or an increase in the proportion of infants who are breast-fed to 75 per cent at birth and 50 per cent at six weeks of age. This approach is to focus right at the very end of the process of health care – on 'outcomes' – but precious little is said about the means (particularly the resources) for achieving these targets, which look so attractively firm on paper. By contrast the Labour Party argues that targets must be matched by action, and thus focuses almost as exclusively on what it will do rather than on where it expects to get to: there are thirty action 'steps' divided into ten priority areas such as child and mental health (make nursery places available to all three- and four-year-olds, reduce the use of tranquillizers), and tobacco and alcohol (ban or control advertising). By contrast, then, this is to focus, at a slightly earlier stage in health care, on 'outputs' rather than 'outcomes', but there are no real concrete targets laid out with which to judge achievements at the very end of the overall process.

The Liberal Democrats, like the Labour Party, show a keen awareness that preventing ill health and promoting good health are matters of broad concern:

> Beveridge saw the NHS as only one part of 'a comprehensive policy of social progress'. It can only be fully effective when it is able to operate within such a policy. A great part of the burden of health care arises from the way in which, separately and collectively, we live our lives. Some of the work of the NHS is preventive medicine, but at present the health service is mainly concerned with the treatment of disease. Social and Liberal Democrats advocate a fundamental shift of emphasis towards health promotion.
>
> (Social and Liberal Democrats 1989c: 5)

In contrast to the government's typical response in terms of an image of precise 'targeting' of very specific issues, they look to broad social and economic inequalities, working environments, and patterns of consumption as the objects of concern here. They recognise the health costs of unemployment and bad housing, and thus the implications for health of policies in these other areas. They commit themselves to an entire ban on tobacco and alcohol promotion, and its increased taxation. They suggest a kind of health audit for policy proposals originating in other policy areas, in order to judge any likely impact on health, and they will tax private concerns whose activities have health consequences.

Charges

A fourth theme which overlaps with earlier issues of funding and prevention is the vexed question of health care charges, in particular prescription charges. The government's strategy has been to raise sharply the level of charges, while operating an extensive exemption mechanism applying to a very substantial minority of the population. The aim is simply to prevent unnecessary use (or at least to dampen demand generated by a very low entry price), and to raise money, albeit not a great deal (about 4 per cent of health care expenditure). The Labour Party expresses great concern about the effects of charges that have been levied on eye tests and dental check-ups, and which they would provide for free (Harman 1992). There is no doubt that there has been a fall in demand for these since charges were introduced which may lead to greater problems (and expenditure) in the future. However, it is unclear what would be done about prescription charges, although the Labour Party is very critical of increases since 1979 (from 20p to £3.40). In their calculations of Labour's expenditure plans the government assumes that there would be a reduction to £2.40 (Conservative Party 1991).

The Social and Liberal Democrats have suggested (SLD 1989c) that they would phase out all charges – not only for prescriptions but also for dental, optical, and ambulance services. They argue that these still deter some patients from seeking proper treatment, constitute an unnecessary increase in administrative work, and undermine the general principle of free health care. They do not address the economic arguments for restraining demand. By

1992, this bold proposal had been reduced to a proposed freeze on charges and an extension of exemptions (Liberal Democrats 1992).

Power

All parties seem concerned about the power of the main professional groups within the NHS. Indeed, the recent history of NHS innovations in the broad view can be characterised as a struggle between state managers and the professions, not least to get greater control over funding decisions, which were traditionally driven by clinical autonomy. The 1991 changes in this respect are merely another (although probably more effective) attempt by the state to introduce structural constraints on professional power – this time through market rather than bureaucratic forces. However, there is a third group with a legitimate interest here, which has traditionally been largely excluded from this titanic struggle – the patients. Attempts to empower the patient have been justified on three grounds: democratic principle, better health, and controlling the professions. The mechanisms of empowerment have followed changes in state control. Thus in the 1970s and 1980s there were bureaucratic mechanisms such as local Community Health Councils and the Health Service Commissioner, while the government now hopes that the Charter and the new quasi-market mechanism will turn patients into consumers, and that money 'attached' to the patient will enforce greater medical responsiveness.

While, like all the parties, it has endorsed the idea of a Charter, the Labour Party is deeply suspicious of the market idea for two reasons. First is the simple point that markets only empower people if they have money. Second, as economists might add, the consumer must also have the information to make informed judgements. In practice these points raise legitimate doubts about the 1991 reforms, because the amount of 'medical money' that is being made available on behalf of each patient by the government may be insufficient to sustain demand for existing services. Moreover this is not directly under the control of the patient, since each District Health Authority decides what health care it will purchase, which may not be what a particular patient wants. This double shortfall will, the Labour Party fears, be topped up in a variety of private ways that will introduce greater inequalities into health care.

In addition to a Charter, the Labour Party is also committed to a no-fault compensation scheme for patients who suffer medical damage so that they will no longer have to prove negligence, thereby saving both legal costs and frustration and anxiety (Cook 1990).

In keeping with their preference for local power, the Liberal Democrats, in addition to their Charter, wish to see much greater local accountability in the NHS. They are no keener on a market than the Labour Party, and this is therefore to be achieved in two alternative ways. First is strengthening community health councils with additional powers and resources. Second, harping back to the Green Paper discussions of the 1960s, they propose either a merging with local government or, should that prove too costly to achieve, they would like to develop direct local accountability either through direct elections or carefully balanced repre-sentation on local NHS management structures (SLD 1989c).

The implications

In sum, the government and the other parties exhibit some curious contrasts in these five areas. Although they seem to be quite bitterly opposed over financial policies, in other areas there is a degree of (often heavily disguised) agreement. On the overall structure of the NHS all are reluctantly in agreement with the idea of splitting strategic and operational management. On patients' rights, policies are almost identical, each party agreeing that a Charter for patients is needed. Similarly, all parties are concerned to curb professional power, and wish to empower patients. However, the mechanisms are quite different, ranging from the market on the one hand to local political accountability on the other. And on the question of future health strategy there are rather complementary analyses, on the one hand concerned with outcomes and on the other with outputs.

What are the implications for resources? We can now return to some of the factors identified earlier in the chapter that any government has to face as having a key bearing on resources. How do the main parties plan to tackle some of these factors?

Most observers see demography and technological develop-ment as two factors that are in reality difficult for any government to do anything about. They give rise to the common assumption that the NHS needs an annual increase of inflation plus 2 per cent merely to stand still in terms of meeting health needs (Robinson and Judge 1987). The Conservative approach is to bear down on health care demand and inefficient resource use using market mechanisms, thereby in their view returning power to the patient as a consumer to top up health care use as desired.

Labour and Liberal Democrat views are united in opposition to this model, accepting that the demographic and technological effects just have to be paid for. The Liberal Democrats, free from the burden of any realistic chance of gaining power, reiterate the point that by international standards the NHS is cheap, and that consequently there is room for expenditure increases as a share of GNP, whatever is happening to economic growth. The Labour Party, quite naturally shy of giving such ammunition to a hostile press, has maintained more prudently that increased expenditure must be paid for in part by increased economic growth.

It is in the other three areas of social, economic and political factors that greater policy choices appear, and where we can detect party disagreements. The Conservative approach to these issues is to avoid the wider (and potentially very expensive) resource implications of tackling social inequality as a general source of illness and poor health care utilisation. Rather, they would wish to target specific conditions and thereby feel justified in ignoring others that are either difficult to specify precisely, or for which it is difficult to tie specific interventions to outcome. Thus, for example, cancer can be ignored, and the issue of tobacco advertising, or industrial pollution, avoided. Similarly, European directives over such advertising can be resisted on the grounds that it is difficult to make unambiguous links to specific outcomes.

The economic and political factors for Conservatives are to be dealt with in the main through the disciplines of the market, since both bureaucratic control of the professions, and consumer representation through local political mechanisms, is felt to be both ineffectual and undesirable.

The Liberal Democrat and Labour Parties accept that wider social inequalities do cause avoidable ill health, and claim to be prepared to spend resources both directly on health care and indirectly on other social measures to try to improve the situation, even if it is difficult to tie specific interventions to specific effects.

As far as the general economic and political factors are

concerned, both opposition parties are concerned about the negative consequences of market mechanisms, either in terms of deterring genuine need or of generating a two-tier service, and are prepared to commit the extra resources necessary to avoid this. For political control, however, their emphases are more inclined towards local and central representation respectively, although they accept that the distinction between strategic planning and detailed management at the heart of the internal market could be continued.

Conservative policy is thus mainly focused on regaining state control over the NHS through target setting, tougher management, and the restructuring of incentives. Liberal Democrat and Labour policy is by contrast focused more on issues of access to a well-funded service, the distribution and nature of illness, control through representative mechanisms, and the conditions of service for NHS staff. While media and political debate contrasts Conservative prudence with Labour and Liberal social concerns, many detailed health policies are common to all three parties.

POLICY OPTIONS FOR THE FUTURE

We can now turn to a discussion of the options available for health policy in the face of both the factors affecting demand for resources, and the current situation within the NHS as it has developed to date. We can distinguish for convenience the short- and medium-term possibilities. In the short term the current state of the NHS, after the 1992 election, has generated debate in three areas: immediate expenditure options, rationing of current demand, and current structural changes. For the medium term, rather than rehearse the range of options reviewed earlier in the inter-party debate, we can examine both the international experience from Europe and North America as an exercise in the art of the possible, and some of the theoretical debates in the health care literature.

Short term

Immediate expenditure options for the NHS are dictated by the current recession which is costing money both in terms of direct social security expenditure, and the loss of government revenues from depressed economic activity. With the public sector borrowing requirement expected to rise to about £30 billion per annum to 1994, there will be very strong pressure from the Treasury to contain public spending in real terms, even if there is no more room for the kind of real cuts that were undertaken in the early 1980s. Given that NHS funds grew quite substantially in the 1990–2 period to cushion the effects of the 1991 restructuring, it is inevitable that this rate of increase must falter. Indeed, it has been commonly observed that even if the government had lost the election, this pattern could not have been avoided in the 1992–4 period (Brindle 1992).

In a situation of growing demand and finite resources, economists predict that prices should rise. In the non-market NHS this takes the form of rationing. This is nicely highlighted by the government's commitment, before the 1992 election, to meet its Patient's Charter right to a maximum of two years' wait for hospital treatment, and the consequent scramble to reduce the backlog of cases amidst criticism of statistical manipulation and purchases from the private sector. In many ways this is politically rather than practically urgent, in that over 90 per cent of cases wait less than a year, about 10 per cent wait one to two years, and very few wait longer. Thus in contrast to the overall budget this commitment will cost relatively little; however, it demonstrates the way in which non-market rather than market rationing can become highly politically charged.

In theory, the scissors of expenditure restraint and politically sensitive rationing in the NHS will be diffused in the 1991 reform, by making the rationing 'disappear' within the 'objective logic' of the market. The 1991 reforms were not all introduced immediately, partly because, as has been widely noted, they have not been tested in advance. Thus only a limited number of trusts and GP budget holders appeared in the first year. The option now is whether to proceed slowly down this path, or to press ahead quickly to avoid getting stuck with a mixed system. General experience in public policy suggests evidence in favour of both paths: speed, it is argued, can carry doubters along before they have time to muster their opposition; on the other hand a slower pace might act as a kind of pilot test and give the expected benefits time to show – particularly if the most favourable cases are the first to convert. The government has shown signs of some uncertainty over this issue of pace, suggesting that it is an area subject to heightened political sensitivity.

These immediate options look less wide than the political rhetoric that appeared at the time of the election might suggest. Even the 1991 reforms have been accepted in part by the other parties, in that both agree that it is sensible to separate strategic planning and detailed management, and influential comment-ators within the field of health policy, such as Chris Ham, have adopted an attitude of wait and see (O'Sullivan 1992). This implicit agreement is an ideal example of what Harrison *et al.* (1990) have termed the 'shared version' in British health policy analysis. They characterise this in terms of nine major features, of which the key ones constitute a system of policy incrementalism through partisan mutual adjustment, in which the medical profession dominates, followed by central and local health managers, with consumers a long way behind. These widely shared analytic assumptions illustrate how difficult it is to think the unthinkable, even for a radical Conservative government.

Medium term

One way of thinking the unthinkable is to turn to the experience of other countries. We can do this in two ways. One is to examine other health care systems for ideas about alternative policies that might be transferable to Britain. The other way is to use a sample of other countries to examine the empirical relationship between health-related variables, such as demand for health care in relation to economic growth. In the space available here we can only give a brief indication of what might be done.

Probably the most common source for alternative ideas for health policy in recent years is the USA (see OECD 1990b for an extensive comparison). Both of the two main innovations in the 1991 reforms have explicit parallels in the USA. GP fund-holders are operating the functional equivalent of American Health Main-tenance Organisations, and trust hospitals operate within parameters similar to those of 'not-for-profit' American hospitals. As such, observers have sought to find evidence with which to both criticise and defend the new structures. The criticisms stem from the weaknesses of the US system, which include the absence of cover for about one-sixth of the population, poor health indicators, and high and rising costs (including administrative costs).

Ironically, it is these very deficiencies in the market that have resulted in the US being the widely acknowledged world leader in health system innovations – necessity being the mother of these inventions. Indeed, it is not only the UK that has turned to the US for ideas: the Netherlands and Germany have adopted similar innovations, and Sweden and France are both looking hard at the benefits that market innovation might bring (Enthoven 1990). However, critics again suggest that these innovations often look attractive only against the backdrop of serious market imperfections, and that by continuing to avoid markets Europe can best retain the superior performance (in terms of health activity and costs) that it already has. Potential gains may carry other heavy prices in terms of market administration, under-provision for the poor, and rapidly rising medical wages. These, it is argued, are worse than the delays and poor choice caused by non-market rationing mechanisms.

In terms of likely real policy options, the bulk of current opinion sees the 1990s as a period of 'new convergence' in health policies in the western world (Reinhardt 1990). The British innovations are not radical by European standards, and many influential American observers recognise that there are many valuable lessons to be learned from the European experience. Enthoven, the architect of the British health reforms, claims that:

> Labour rhetoric notwithstanding, there is no prospect for the Europeans to adopt the American system or vice versa. And there is no point in discussing whose system is superior. The really interesting questions are how to identify and design politically feasible incremental changes in each country that have a reasonably good chance of making things better. Each country can get useful ideas from others about how to do this.
> (Enthoven 1990: 58)

The second way to use the experience of other countries is to take a sample of industrial countries – usually the OECD set – and examine the pattern of associated variables in them. The simplest method is to take a dependent variable such as the total proportion and changes in it of gross national product spent on health care in total, or by the state, and try to find out what factors, of the sort discussed in the first part of this chapter, can best explain the variation in it. An example is provided by Culyer (1990) with data on OECD countries for the period 1960–84. He discovers that the main factors that explain the rise in health care expenditure in different countries (and hence the best guide to policy options aimed at squaring the circle for this particular policy area) are income per capita, utilisation (population changes plus technology), and the extent of private ownership of health services; limits on expenditure are associated with central budgeting and public financing. However, in thinking about the policy implications of the data, Culyer concludes:

> The selective use of instruments that appear to bear on these components currently offers the best way forward: promoting competition between suppliers, use of closed-ended prospective systems for paying suppliers, controlling entry to the major professional groups, use of salary and capitation rather than fee for service in medical remuneration, and various direct price and volume controls. None is a panacea and none is without its own cost.
>
> (Culyer 1990: 39)

CONCLUSION

What does all this add up to in terms of our understanding of the demand for health care? Traditionally the answer should be framed in terms of specific theoretical assumptions. For much of this chapter we have accepted the self-understanding of governments and political parties about what might be possible 'in the given circumstances'. This has given rise to the idea of 'managed competition' – a 'new convergence' between the twin poles of state and market through a kind of 'public contract' in which state agencies represent the public in the collective purchase of health care from a variety of separate and competing suppliers. This, it is hoped, will combine the efficiencies of macro-level budgetary control and micro-level market efficiency. Theoretically, this is very close to the idea of Harrison *et al.* (1990), already referenced, that there is a common (-sense) view or 'shared version' of health policy. Elsewhere I have argued at length why this approach in social policy is wrong (Manning 1985: Ch. 7), on the grounds that the analysis is distorted by ideology. Harrison *et al.* also challenge this common-sense view, and lay out the grounds for adequate theory in this field which they try to meet drawing on neo-élite and neo-marxist theories, because they feel that 'despite some consonances, the "shared version" is not sufficiently consistent with the events of the last decade to constitute an adequate explanation' (Harrison *et al.* 1990: 153).

A case study of the 'shared version' is provided by Salter (1992) in a study of the Medway District Health Authority in Kent as it tries to put the new NHS structures into practice. Salter argues that far from an integrated package, 'managed competition' contains irresolvable contradictions between central state directives and locally generated demands and priorities. It is thus ideological, in my terms (Manning 1985), in that it is a model of what certain groups would wish to occur, but which in fact hides the reality of the structures and policy dynamics that are actually evolving, for example, the recent breakdown in NHS dental services, and the seeming rapid escalation of privatisation in this part of the NHS. Policy development and implementation are, in fact, inherently contestable political processes, as much of this book serves to show.

Chapter 8

The personal social services
The politics of care

John Baldock

The future of the local authority personal social services has never been a central issue in British general elections. This was as true in 1992 as before. Similarly, debate and legislation about social service issues has rarely excited much attention in the House of Commons. Phoebe Hall, in her book about the political process that accompanied the legislation to implement the Seebohm Report, one of the more substantial reforms of personal social services in the post-war era, tells how the minister responsible, Richard Crossman, regarded the effort as 'boring', that the Labour cabinet found the report 'contemptible' and that 'the proposals were non-contentious in a party-political sense . . . the debates were poorly attended and they lacked the sparkle of other legislation' (Hall 1976: 82, 83, 107).

This is to some extent because the detail of personal social service provision is a local government matter. Party conflict on social service issues in the county and metropolitan councils can some-times be bitter and intense. Formally it is they who decide how much shall be spent each year on their social services but they do so within expenditure and policy constraints which are set by central government and which rarely allow them much room for man-oeuvre. There is a large and complex literature about how much local party politics affects levels of service provision (Sharpe and Newton 1984; Barnett *et al.* 1990). While there is some evidence that Labour-controlled councils spend more on social services, inter-pretation is made difficult by the fact that Labour are more likely to be the dominant party in authorities with greater social needs. Some 80 per cent of the money available to local councils comes from or is directly determined by central government. Much of it is allocated on the basis of an elaborate 'standard spending assessment' using indicators of need which have frequently been questioned as being partial and arbitrary (Derbyshire 1987; DoE 1987b). The issue has been further complicated in recent years by the introduction of charge- and expenditure-capping which severely limit the room for local political discretion. Central government makes the essential decisions determining how much money will be available for the personal social services. But it makes them with only a broad and technical reference to social need. It also decides the duties and objectives of the services. Local authorities must do the best they can to fulfil their legal obligations within the funds made available to them. They can usually only spend more on one service by cutting another. In this sense, this is an area of social policy where national government does not have to square the circle. They do not have to limit their policies to what can be 'afforded', nor do they have to take much account of scale of need.

The theme of this chapter is that needs play a surprisingly small part in determining the scale and scope of the personal social services. Need, in the sense of numbers of people and their circumstances, is just one of the factors that decide personal social services provision. There are many other, often more important, ingredients in the mix: changes in professional opinion and behaviour, decisions about local government organisation and finance, developments in other parts of the welfare system such as in housing and health services, press outcry when the negligent, cruel or unacceptable is discovered. The processes which determine the evolution of the personal social services are very political, perhaps more so than in other, more overtly politicised areas of social policy, such as social security, education and the National Health Service. In those much larger services substantial proportions of provision are demand-led: the more people in the relevant categories, the greater public expenditure. In contrast, in the case of the personal social services it is quite common for local authorities, their choices squeezed between expenditure- and charge-capping, to decide to reduce levels of real expenditure in the face of growing need.

NEED, DEMAND AND SUPPLY OF THE PERSONAL SOCIAL SERVICES

None the less, debate about the future of the personal social services continues to be couched in terms of needs. There is a shared convention that the publicly-funded personal social services exist to help the most frail and vulnerable in our society. Politicians, professionals and public all find it more comfortable to use the language of need. So too does the major legislation governing the services. Two key pieces of legislation will dominate the development of local authority personal social services in the 1990s: Part III of the NHS and Community Care Act 1990 and the Children Act 1989. Both acts require local authorities to monitor and to meet need. The Children Act requires that authorities 'take reasonable steps to identify the extent to which there are children in need within their area' and specifies categories of relevant need. The community care legislation goes further, asking authorities to produce annual figures of the numbers in their communities likely to require services and to submit plans to the Secretary of State indicating how they propose to meet that need. The whole tenor of the legislation sustains the well-established fiction that in some way the provision of local authority social services is proportionate to need.

In fact, there are few reasons to expect that in the 1990s the supply of services will or can respond directly to changes in social need. Were they to do so it would amount to a reversal of past experience. Whereas it is reasonable to consider how health, education and social security services have grown or shrunk in relation to need, such a question is rather less meaningful when asked of the personal social services. Local authority social services have rarely been sufficient to offer assistance to more than a minority of those likely to be defined as in need of help. This is not in itself a criticism of the level of provision. There are good reasons for arguing that the state should seek to provide only a proportion of the care of dependent people. The point is that once this has been accepted it makes no sense to look for or expect clear correlations between measures of need and the supply of public services.

It is worth rehearsing a few figures which indicate how loose is the link between need and the volume of public personal social services. If one selects any dimension of need central to the work of social services departments, one finds that only a small proportion of the relevant population is receiving help. For example, the elderly, particularly the very frail, are the group most likely to be in contact with local authority social services. We know that just over half of people aged 85 and older who are still living in the community are effectively house-bound and unable to perform household tasks or do their own shopping. Yet less than 36 per cent of this age group receive the home help service and most of those get two hours or less a week, 11 per cent get meals on wheels and only 6 per cent attend a day centre (OPCS 1989a). Even these national figures mean little, so great is the variation in the supply of services between authorities. For example, the supply of home help hours in Derbyshire is 400 per cent greater per head of population over the age of 85 than it is in Surrey (DoH 1990).

At the other end of the age spectrum one might consider provision for disabled children living in the community. A national survey in the mid-1980s found that amongst those with the most severe disabilities, effectively those requiring constant attention, only 2 per cent had seen a social worker in the last year although 24 per cent of the parents said they needed the help of a social worker (OPCS 1989b: Tables 4.12, 4.21). Again, the variation in child-care services between authorities is enormous: for example, day-care provision in Buckinghamshire is nearly five times as generous as in South Tyneside (DoH 1990). The effective consequence for users is that 'these variations turn their access to services into a game of geographical chance' (Harding 1992).

Most of the mentally ill in the community have no contact with local authority social services; neither do a majority of people who are blind or partially-sighted (Mental Health Foundation 1990; RNIB 1991). Similar examples could be repeated almost *ad infinitum* for every area of need for which local authority services are nominally responsible; rarely are more than a tiny minority of the relevant group known to the social services (see Hunter and Wistow 1991; DoH 1991a; Evandrou *et al.* 1990).

Further confirmation of the lack of any direct linkage between need and the supply of public personal social services is provided by making international comparisons. Differences in services, variety of organisational forms, and accounting practices make such comparisons crude, but the variations in the amounts of service supplied are so large that they overwhelm these technical difficulties. For example, one study estimated that health and social care expenditure per person over 75 in 1985 varied between £950 per head in England to over £4,000 per head in the Netherlands. It was also found that the provision of home help hours was over four times as great relative to population in Sweden as it was in England (Kraan *et al.* 1991: 234–5).

It is well established that the vast amount of care work not done by the state is provided by families and, to a lesser extent, informally within local communities. It is equally well accepted that the nature of the family as a caring organisation is in flux and under threat (Finch 1989; Kiernan and Wicks 1990). Politicians and policy analysts have realised that quite small reductions in the supply of family care could have substantial costs for the public sector if it had to fill the gap (Audit Commission 1992). Governments have sometimes sought to limit the damage that an explosion of pent-up demand might do to personal social service budgets by arguing that the provision of services should grow in line with changes in numbers in the main need groups. This approach of course ignores the obvious point that this is only a convincing position if service levels start from some justifiable match with needs. None the less, it is a political expedient which has served governments well, first emerging in a clear way under the last Labour government after the sterling crisis of 1976. In order to keep within the public expenditure and borrowing limits set by the International Monetary Fund it became necessary to 'cash limit' much of public expenditure. The government issued a white paper indicating how spending on the health and social services could be contained and yet match the changes in needs produced by demographic growth (DHSS 1976). The document suggested, without much substantiation, that a figure of about 2 per cent real growth in service provision per year would be necessary to keep up with demographic factors. This guideline has, over time, become institutionalised into an accepted bench-mark around which debate about the right levels of provision has tended to be conducted.

Demographic change in an industrial society is very gradual and so the argument that public services should match it is often a very conservative one. Consider, for example, some of the population changes in the 1990s that might be expected to affect, for want of a more exact term, fundamental need for social service provision. Between 1991 and 2001 the UK population is predicted to grow by 3.3 per cent. The two largest population groups relevant to the personal social services are children – numbers under age 15 will grow by 6.3 per cent – and the old – numbers aged 75 and over will grow by 5.6 per cent. The number of households, the basic social unit with which social services have to deal, will grow by 3.8 per cent, slightly faster than the population. The faster rate of growth in households is due almost entirely to the fact that more people of all ages are for one reason or another finding themselves living in smaller units, and particularly on their own. Single-person households will increase by 21.8 per cent in the period. Although by far the largest number of people living on their own are people over the age of retirement, and this group will increase by 30 per cent over the period, it is amongst people of working age that the rate of growth of single-person households is fastest. This is because of both delayed marriage and increased divorce. The number of 30–44-year-olds living on their own will grow by over 100 per cent. Rising numbers of divorces and separations will also largely account for the expected increase in the number of single-parent families, a rise of 6 per cent during the period (data taken from DoE 1988; OPCS 1989c).

While it is difficult to draw easy conclusions from gross figures of expected population growth, there does appear to be a clear prospect that those categories of household that are more likely to require social service help are growing at a faster rate than the overall population. However, the rates of increase even of key groups such as the very old and children are such that, all other things remaining equal, real increases in expenditure of less than 1 per cent a year can be argued to be sufficient to keep pace.

None the less, the idea that governments can be held to account against some notional, population-based figure has become a political force in its own right, a minimal test of whether the circle has been squared. Lately, it seems, government wishes to escape even this criterion. For many years the MPs on the House of Commons Social Services Committee have questioned ministers and civil servants responsible for provision in the area using the 'benchmark figure of 2 per cent growth as necessary to keep up with demographic and other factors' (House of Commons 1991: para 107). Yet in 1991 the Health Committee of the Commons, the successor to the old Social Services Committee, discovered even this could no longer be relied upon:

> We asked officials from the Department of Health how the figure of 2 per cent growth was calculated. To our surprise Mr Luce, Under Secretary in the Department's Community Services Division, told us: ' . . . the department has never used an overall PSS growth benchmark figure of the 2 per cent kind.

. . . At times in the past I think the Committee have been told or formed the view that tended to get to an overall figure of about 2 per cent but I do want to emphasise that only the demography element in that is precisely calculable, and the rest is a much more general assessment'.

(House of Commons 1991: para 108)

The Committee's report went on to demonstrate that the 2 per cent figure was no figment of their imagination but had indeed been used by the department quite frequently in the past. They then recommended 'that the government publish each year in the Department's Annual Report its estimates of the amount needed to meet demographic and other pressures, and that the various components of the sum should be separately identified and quantified' (1991: para 110).

The Department of Health's response, in its 1992 report, was to produce an analysis of expected growth in demand for the hospital and community health services that shows demographic factors (age groups weighted in proportion to their current use of services) growing at rates of between 0.5 per cent and 0.9 per cent a year between 1990 and 1998 (DoH and OPCS 1992). These, rather unalarming, estimates of the effect of demographic forces are similar to those described by social demographers. Discussing the effects of an ageing population, John Ermisch has argued, 'even if we look 40 years ahead (to 2026), expenditures on health and personal social services would only need to be 12 per cent higher if the expenditure per person in each age group were maintained at its 1986–87 level' (Ermisch 1990: 43). However, it should be borne in mind that all 'future-need' calculations of this sort are based on methodologies that can be debated and on assumptions about future numbers that may well be wrong. These problems apply especially when discussing the populations most relevant to the personal social services: the very old and the very young.

Both future births and future deaths are subject to a degree of uncertainty. On one hand, 'forecasting future fertility is the most difficult task in demography, and seldom successfully attempted' (Coleman and Salt 1992: 145). The decision to have children is affected by a huge range of factors, economic, social and psychological, and the size and even direction of these factors change over time. In particular, it has proved very difficult to

forecast the changes in the fortunes of the economy which appear
to be central in determining fertility. Demographers are, on the
whole, unable to predict short-term blips in the fertility rate such
as the abrupt fall to 1977 and the sharp rise since 1987.
Consequently, the social services get fairly short notice of relevant
changes in the numbers of young children. On the other hand,
predicting the numbers of old people is, perhaps surprisingly, also
very difficult. Over the last decade the OPCS has regularly found
it necessary to revise expected mortality rates downwards as
longevity has steadily increased. For example, the prediction of
the number of pensioners by 2011 has risen by over 9 per cent
since the 1979-based projection (Craig 1983).

It also makes a considerable difference when allowance is made
for the fact that service use (and presumably need) increases
amongst the elderly with age. It is currently expected that the size
of the retired population will fall by just over 1 per cent between
1991 and 2001 (OPCS 1989c). This is due to the lower birth rates
in the 1920s and early 1930s. Fewer people will be joining the
ranks of the retired over the next decade. However, this means
that the proportion of the retired in the older age cohorts will rise.
In the DoH estimates of need, retired people are weighted in
three age groups: 60/65–74, 75–84 and 85 and over (DoH and
OPCS 1992: Fig. 6). Between 1991 and 2001 the age cohort
60/65–74 falls markedly, the 75–84 cohort is stable but the 85+
cohort will grow between 20 per cent and 25 per cent depending
on the course of mortality rates. The weighting used can therefore
make a crucial difference to need estimates. The demographer
John Craig has considered a number of service use indicators
(institutionalisation, use of home helps, being an in-patient, and
mortality) and these rise by factors of between 5 and 10 when the
over 80s are compared with those 20 years younger. By applying
weighting based on these indicators, Craig shows how the
population over retirement age between 1991 and 2001, instead
of falling as the crude numbers indicate, will rise by up to 18 per
cent in terms of current levels of service use (Craig 1983).

We have concentrated on the links between personal social
service provision and demographic measures of need because
these are the terms in which most significant political debate is
conducted. That public debate is limited in this way is in itself a
political achievement. None of the major political parties appear
anxious to include other more social factors in the calculus of

need. In contrast, within the social service community of professionals and researchers, it is widely accepted that a far more important determinant of need than relatively slow demographic changes is the scale of poverty in the community.

> The most striking characteristics that clients of the personal social services have in common are poverty and deprivation. Often this is not mentioned, possibly because social services are said to be based on universalistic principles. Still, everyone in the business knows it . . . as many as 80 per cent (of clients) have incomes at or below income support levels.
>
> (Schorr 1992: 8)

It is not that those with higher incomes do not suffer the problems that the personal social services are formally there to help with: disability, dependence, family strife and child care problems. They do, but the chances that they will seek or obtain help from local authority social services departments is slight. The fundamental, but largely unwritten, rationing rule applied by the services is that those who can pay for help elsewhere should do so. The result is that the public service is one of last resort and the effective determinants of demand for them are the causes of poverty: unemployment, particularly long-term, low pay, low benefits and homelessness. As these change, so does 'need' for the personal social services.

For the past decade all these social sources of need have risen far more than the marginal shifts in the demographic indices that are the basis of authoritative political debate. At the time of writing (late 1992) there seems little likelihood that Britain will in the rest of the 1990s enjoy an economic revival sufficient to change these trends. However, this chapter will not explore in greater depth the ways in which what has been called the 'poverty complex' of low incomes, unemployment, old age and homelessness generates need because these are not the conventional terms of inter-party political debate. There seems to exist almost a cartel of silence amongst national politicians on this issue. While they will sometimes debate, say, unemployment and homelessness as discrete issues, they also seem to agree that it would be committing too many hostages to fortune to admit that when governments fail in these areas they should be ready to spend more on the personal social services.

Thus, although the politicians on the Commons Health Committee may find it politically effective to require governments to justify social expenditures in terms of demographic change, this can only be the first step in indicating how provision should respond. It is simply the case that the provision of public personal social services is only very slightly a consequence of the scale of social need in a community. Services are far too small to allow the conclusion that if they grow in line with population, however weighted, they are thereby growing with need. There is already a sufficient gap between provision and any reliable measure of need to justify multiplying the level of public personal social services several times over. The local authority social services not only face substantial increases in need over the next decade; they also start from the position of a very substantial, if largely unmeasured, gap between needs and service supply. The 'needs–supply gap' constitutes a permanent potential for a rapid increase in demand for the services.

THE POLITICS OF PERSONAL SOCIAL SERVICES EXPENDITURE

The local authority social services departments have enjoyed two periods of substantial real growth: 1971 to 1976 and 1986 to 1992. In the first period expenditure grew at a compound rate of nearly 14 per cent. It then fell to just over 2 per cent per year. Between 1986 and 1992 the rate accelerated again to nearly 6 per cent a year allowing for changes in prices (Table 8.1). However, these national figures hide enormous variations between authorities, some growing much faster than the overall national figure, some actually contracting. For example, amongst the authorities in England, between 1984/5 and 1990/1, of 107 authorities, 30 increased real expenditure by 40 per cent or more, 67 by between 10 per cent and 39 per cent, seven by between zero and 9 per cent and three reduced expenditure, one of which did so by more than 5 per cent (House of Commons 1991: Table 22.7). This spread is due to a wide variety of factors, some of which are the product of local politics, others the result of central government rules about rate- and charge-capping.

However, spending by local authorities on the work of the social services departments is really only part of the tale. The pressure of demand has found other ways to express itself. In particular, the overall costs to the state of funding the demographically-driven expansion in community care have grown through relatively unplanned and uncontrolled increases

Table 8.1 Real government expenditure on the personal social services
(UK)

	£m (1987/8 prices) [1]	Year on year % increase	Index of real spending (1973/4 = 100)
1973/4	2,478	–	100
1974/5	2,875	16.0	116
1975/6	3,202	11.4	129
1976/7	3,266	1.9	132
1977/8	2,839	−13.1	115
1978/9	2,922	2.9	118
1979/80	3,132	7.2	126
1980/1	3,304	5.5	133
1981/2	3,266	−1.2	132
1982/3	3,300	1.0	133
1983/4	3,408	3.3	138
1984/5	3,460	1.5	140
1985/6	3,783	9.3	153
1986/7	3,974	5.0	160
1987/8	3,856	−3.0	156
1988/9	4,050	5.0	163
1989/90	4,141	2.2	167
1990/1	4,504	8.8	181
1991/2[2]	4,819	7.0	194

Sources: Evandrou *et al.* 1990, Table 6.2; CSO 1992a, Table 3.4; Cm 1913 1992
Notes: [1] GDP deflator; [2] 1991/2 = estimated out-turn

in social security expenditure. The best known of these was the
growth in public funding of people in private and voluntary
residential care through the income support system. Between
1979 and 1992 this expenditure increased from practically zero to
nearly £2 billion a year (Bottomley 1992), paying in whole or in
part for some 150,000 residents at any one time. One result has
been a slight increase in the proportion of elderly people who are
dealing with their care needs by entering an institution rather
than remaining in the community (Laing 1991: Fig. 2). This was
a policy that began almost by accident and was, in part, a
consequence of restrictions on local authority expenditure:

In 1974 local authorities paid for about 60 per cent of voluntary
sector residents in England. By 1983 it had dropped to 34 per
cent. Then they started to look for an alternative source of
money and found it in the Social Security system. Responding
to pressure orchestrated and articulated by voluntary

organisations, local DHSS Social Security offices started to pay supplementary benefits to people unable to afford their own fees, and for whom local authorities were unwilling to foot the bill. Initially there was no national policy . . . but the practice became so widespread that policy was formalised in 1983.

(Laing 1991: 5)

The social security system also funds people in need of personal care through a wide range of direct benefits, and these too have grown in a demand-determined way during the 1980s. The Attendance Allowance was created in 1971 and is payable to those who need either frequent attention or continual supervision. In the first year it was received by 54,000 people. Now more than 800,000 receive it during a year at a cost in 1988–9 of £880 million (House of Commons 1991: Table 17.1; DSS 1991a). The Invalid Care Allowance was introduced in 1976 and is a benefit for those providing regular and substantial care, for thirty-five hours per week or more, to someone receiving the Attendance Allowance. By 1989 it was claimed by over 120,000 people in a typical week and cost £150 million in 1988–9 (Housse of Commons 1991; DSS 1991a). There has also been considerable growth in payments to people in the community who are also eligible for income support: disability premiums, severe disability premiums and pensioner premiums. In addition, dependent people on Income Support have had two other discretionary sources of help: the community care grants provided by the Social Fund (£30 million a year in 1988–9) and, until it was abruptly shut down in November 1992, the Independent Living Fund (£72 million in 1991–2).

In 1988–9 all these forms of social security expenditure on personal care, largely non-existent or negligible before 1980, amounted to at least an additional £2,000 million on top of local authority expenditure that year of £3,406 million. They are an outstanding example of how public funding for personal social services has expanded more through political accident than by design. Expenditure has not grown evenly but has tended to shift abruptly upwards when governments, due to 'political error', have let the demand cat briefly escape from the rationing bag. Because of the needs–supply gap, the capacity for people to use the services is effectively infinite and the capacity of service professionals to find work to do is unlimited. There is always a potential for rapid growth, a 'problem' exacerbated, from the point of view of central government, by the fact that its control of expenditure in this area is indirect, dependent on decisions made by local authorities. The rest of this chapter will consider governments' records in resisting demand for expansion of the personal social services and will go on to speculate about possible developments in the 1990s.

Both the 1960s and the 1980s were periods when government addressed fundamental questions about 'which social welfare services to make available, to whom and how' (Hall 1976: 1) and as a consequence ended those decades by passing legislation substantially changing the goals and organisation of the personal social services. Both the 1970s and the 1990s are periods when the fruits of that legislation become apparent. The earlier legislation, almost unwittingly, opened the floodgates of demand and recent acts can be seen as attempts to close them. To some extent the Conservatives' Community Care Act of 1990 seeks to reverse the consequences of Labour's Social Services Act of 1970. Yet at the time the 1970 Act received little criticism from the Conservative opposition which a few months later found itself overseeing its implementation. Similarly, the two opposition parties did not attack the 1990 reforms in any fundamental way, despite the fact that they contradicted many of their previously avowed principles.

The Social Services Act of 1970 was technically no more than a structural reorganisation of local authority personal social services and involved no explicit resource commitments. However, it laid the foundations for a rapid expansion of public funding. This was what its supporters intended and what government was too distracted to prevent (Parker 1970: 111–12). Thus began a profession-led attempt at a 'comprehensive social service . . . available to all . . . [with] no uncertainty about where to turn for help nor any ambiguity about where responsibility for providing assistance lies' (Seebohm Committee 1968: para 146).

The 1980s might be characterised as the decade in which the Conservatives sought to assert greater central control over the local authority social services and to find a clear rationale for policy. More explicit justifications for a residual service began to emerge. The public personal social services were to be 'a long stop for the very special needs going beyond the range of voluntary service' (Jenkin 1980). Their function was 'to back up and develop the assistance which is given by private and voluntary support'

(Fowler 1984). The need for a policy framework more in keeping with the reality of a marginal service was, implicitly at least, a problem for the opposition parties too. But, as has been pointed out already, there is little political incentive for politicians out of power to concern themselves with the personal social services. When the Labour Party lost power in 1979 it had barely begun to recognise the implications for local social services of the tight control on public expenditure it had instituted. Traditionally, almost unconsciously, the Labour Party still subscribed to a universalist conception of a 'fifth social service' available to all in need in the same way as education or health care. By the end of the 1980s such an implicit conception had melted away. The Labour opposition was criticising the government for delays in carrying out the recommendations of Sir Roy Griffiths (Griffiths 1988), but chose not to dwell on the reality that those reforms placed selectivity and a minimalist conception of the local social services at their very heart.

The Conservative government was forced in the 1980s to grapple with the practical problems which had allowed the Audit Commission to conclude that community care policies were 'in some disarray' and that, unless substantial reform was initiated, a 'window of opportunity to establish an effective community-based service' would be lost. A new policy logic was constructed and the 1990s will test whether their new and radical policies can be made to work. The Conservative government are overseeing a revolution in the way in which public personal social services are provided, a revolution of its own making but one which it is introducing with some reluctance. The Griffiths Report was not particularly to the government's liking. While the report had made a strong case for a mixed economy of welfare in which public responsibilities would no longer be open-ended, it did so by recommending a lead role for local authorities and the transfer of a substantial proportion of central government finance to them. The government took nearly two years to respond to these politically unpalatable suggestions. There is little doubt that Prime Minister Margaret Thatcher and other senior Tories used the time to search, unsuccessfully, for an alternative to increasing the powers and resources of local government. There was further delay when the implementation of the Griffiths reforms was put off because of the political and financial problems of the community charge.

The 1990s will see the implementation of social policies that make it clear that community care is not 'the prerogative of public services' (Departments of Health, Social Security, Wales and Scotland 1989: para 2.21) and that the role of social service departments is that of 'enabling authorities ... securing the delivery of services, not simply by acting as direct providers, but by developing their purchasing and contracting role to become enabling authorities' (1989: para 3.1.3) in a world in which 'the reality is that most care is provided by family, friends and neighbours' (1989: para 2.3). The emphasis is no longer on a universalist concept of a 'fifth social service' but on selective 'services that concentrate on those with the greatest needs' (1989: para 1.10) and which 'make maximum possible use of private and voluntary providers' (1989: para 1.11). The local authority social service departments have entered the 1990s with the need to pursue very different objectives to those that dominated the previous twenty years.

THE DIFFERENCES BETWEEN THE PARTIES

The fact that the Conservative Party has been in government continuously since 1979 has obliged it to be explicit in its intentions. Furthermore, its commitment to policy goals can be tested against what has happened. The two main opposition parties, on the other hand, have been able to take advantage of the low political salience of personal social service issues to leave their policy intentions relatively vague. These are often little more than untestable expressions of goodwill. Certainly neither opposition party has had to face up directly to what might be called the secret conundrum of the personal social services: how to decide the level and direction of a service that in practice meets only a fraction of its potential demand and obligations?

As a result it is not possible to evaluate the differences between the parties along the dimensions used in the other chapters in this book: the balance struck between universal and selective services and between satisfying minimum needs and using a service to undermine inequalities; the positioning of the public–private divide; the emphasis on consumer choice and participation; and the approach to organisational and managerialist problems. This is not because these issues are unimportant but rather because, in the case of the personal social services, the parties have not adopted noticeably different stances. As the rest of this section will seek to show, the two opposition parties have found it difficult to keep up with the radical initiatives of the Conservative government in the last three areas while joining it in a studious silence about the first two. It is arguable that the personal social services, particularly the care of the dependent in the community, have been at the cutting edge of innovative social policy in recent years. The use and encouragement of non-state provision has been made the core of policy, consumer choice has ostensibly been made paramount in deciding what shall be provided, and the consequent organisational reform has produced something close to a state of continuous managerial turmoil (Schorr 1992: 44). Critics have argued that these changes are essentially aimed at ensuring a minimalist and highly selective public provision (Wistow and Henwood 1991; Phillipson 1992). While this may be so, the failure of either the Conservative government or the Labour and Liberal Democrat Parties even to begin to debate the resource implications of the dramatic policy changes has left the argument open. This vagueness is just another example of the fact that, from the point of view of national politics at least, there is no need to square the circle of welfare needs and expenditure constraints.

The Conservative manifesto of 1992 gave more space to personal social service issues than did those of either of the two opposition parties. The policy of the Tories in this area in the 1990s will be largely the implementation of the substantial legislation they have already enacted. There is little recognition in policy documents or in ministerial pronouncements of a response to criticisms of the new policies. In particular, the present Conservative government is giving no quarter to those who argue that a considerable increase in overall funding will be necessary. For example, in an article on policy intentions published just before the 1992 election, the then junior minister responsible for social services, later to become Secretary of State for Health, Virginia Bottomley, stated very specifically that

the policy of community care will be adequately resourced. We are committed to transferring to local government the money we would have spent on social security under the existing system. The transfer from social security will be made explicit showing how the sums are done.

(Bottomley 1992: 19–20)

She indicates that increases in this amount will be made only at

> the rate at which local authorities will assume responsibility for new clients, taking into account demographic and other pressures .... The extra comes only if overall national economic policy is prudent and geared for long-term growth. Government needs a firm idea of priorities.
>
> (Bottomley 1992: 19–20)

At the time of writing, after difficult negotiations between the local authorities and central government over just how much money is to be transferred to finance the new policies from April 1993, a figure of some £530 million has been announced and was greeted by social service managers with relief because it ended uncertainty, but with concern that it will be insufficient.

Labour and the Liberal Democrats have found themselves in the somewhat odd but comfortable position of being able to chide the government for its reluctance and delay in pursuing its own policies. What is hidden by this debate is the fact that the opposition parties have essentially come round to an acceptance of the government's plans and have proposed few alternatives. The conversion of the Conservative Party to 'making a reality of community care' has been a hard and public one. In contrast, the conversion of the opposition parties to the reality of highly selective and harshly rationed services, arguably a far more radical and inconsistent shift in commitments than the Conservatives have had to endure, has taken place in a quiet, hidden, and largely unargued and implicit way.

This is particularly so in the case of the Labour Party. The path it has followed from its 1960s commitments (to an ideal of services determined to seek out unmet need and provide universal provision) to its 1990s realism (acceptance of tightly rationed and often privately provided services) is largely an unmarked route. We do not know how, ideologically and in terms of policy analysis, they have arrived where they are. This is partly because issues about the personal social services are not high on the vote-winning agenda but is also a reflection of Labour's historical ambivalence towards this whole area. The party has never been particularly comfortable with the provision of social work services to individuals. Indeed, historically part of the very *raison d'être* of the Labour Party is the pursuit of policies that would make public personal social services almost unnecessary. The post-war welfare state was constructed by the Attlee government to provide families with incomes sufficient to choose how to solve their personal problems themselves and the homes in which to do so. There is a deep strand in Labour Party ideology, though one that is rarely explicitly articulated these days, that regards the need for personal social services as an indicator of the failure of social policy.

What are the explicit policies of the three main political parties and how do they differ?

As has already been pointed out, the detail of Conservative policy is to be found in the considerable body of personal social service legislation passed in recent years. The only new Conservative policies announced for the personal social services in the 1992 election and in the Queen's speech that followed the re-election of the Conservative Party were:

1 'Additional funding' for voluntary organisations involved in the provision of social care.
2 A requirement that local authorities produce Local Childcare Plans setting out available services.
3 The continuation of the Independent Living Fund, a cash-limited discretionary fund that makes individualised payments to people with disabilities.

The government has also appointed a commission to report on reorganisation of local government. There is a distinct possibility that the existing two-tier system across much of the country may be replaced by a single level. If this does occur, it will mean, just as it did in 1974, that the social services departments will be plunged into further organisational turmoil before they have had time to adjust to their own internal transformation.

At the time of the 1992 election, Labour had proposed:

1 Renaming to create the 'Department of Health and Community Care' and the appointment of a Minister of State for Community Care. These were both recommended by the Griffiths Report and designed to give personal social service issues a higher profile in a central government ministry traditionally preoccupied with running the health service.
2 Earmarking that part of central government's grant to the local authorities which was intended for expenditure on the personal social services, thus preventing underspending

compared with the levels assumed in the standard expenditure assessments. While the Conservatives initially resisted this 'ring-fencing', they have agreed to it on a temporary basis as from April 1993.

3 Improving and extending the Invalid Care Allowance 'as resources allow'. This presumably referred to discussion in previous policy documents about the creation of a 'carer's benefit' which would be paid, as the present Invalid Care Allowance is not, to carers over retirement age (Cook 1990; Blunkett 1991). This is the largest group of carers, mainly spouses caring for each other, and the extension of the care allowance to them, without a reduction in other benefits, would amount to a major development in the system of community care.

4 Creating equality in the public funding arrangements for local authority residential homes and private homes, thus preventing the need for local authorities to 'privatise' their homes. Conservative policy has made it uneconomic for local authorities to continue running their own residential homes.

5 Setting up a 'Quality Commission', incorporating the present Audit Commission and linked to a system of independent locally-based inspectors, to monitor local services together with clear arrangements for citizens to complain and get redress.

6 Improving the predictability of local authority funding of the voluntary sector by introducing a system where three-year grants become the usual model for core funding.

Amongst the specific promises that the Labour Party did not make in the 1992 election but might have been expected to make were: ending the expenditure capping by central government that prevents some local authorities spending as much as they would like on the personal social services; and implementation of sections 1–3 of the Disabled Persons Act 1986 requiring public funding of an independent advocacy service.

Overall, Labour appear to have been careful to make few specific promises in the area of the personal social services but to stick to more vague talk of developing 'a high quality programme of community care which responds to what users want' and of local authorities returning 'to the centre stage in making the right kind of care available through the development of innovative domiciliary and respite provision' (Blunkett 1991: 4.14).

However, a Labour government would probably have its greatest effect on the amount and nature of personal social services not through policies which deal directly with them but through the consequences of other areas of social policy. As has already been pointed out, there is a core of Labour ideology that sees personal provision as demeaning and unnecessary. Central to Labour's promises has always been a commitment to minimise social need by reducing unemployment and raising social security benefits. In the 1992 election the party promised to raise Child Benefit and pensions above the levels intended by the existing government and to tie the state pension to increases in earnings where these were higher than the rise in prices. A similar policy on pensions through the 1980s would have left the basic pension 20 per cent higher and kept many more retired people out of income support. Another of the more expensive promises Labour made was to rapidly expand nursery education for 3- and 4-year-olds until places were available for all children who wanted them by the end of the century. It is impossible to quantify the income effects of these changes, let alone their consequences for the volume of need for personal social services amongst dependent people and families with children. In principle, the provision of greater resources, particularly income, to allow people to deal with their own needs should reduce demand on the personal social services. But, as has been pointed out, the existing gap between need and supply is already so huge as to make an observable effect most unlikely. This allows the paradoxical conclusion that Labour's policies might even be bad for the personal social services in so far as increased public expenditure on the core and expensive parts of the welfare state – social security, hospital care, education and housing – might draw resources away from the social services. There is no doubt that in Labour's welfare policies there are to be found at least the remnants of its traditional preference for universal, often cash-based, forms of provision. This is a conception of social welfare which leaves the needs- and means-tested local authority social services until last.

There are other parts of Labour's avowed policies where the indirect consequences for the personal social services might be more positive. In 1992 the party proposed, if elected, to create a Ministry for Women represented at cabinet level. It has long been pointed out that most work of the social services is with or through women so such a development would surely raise awareness of needs in the personal social services. Similarly, Labour's promise of a 'Charter of Rights' backed by legislation specifying 'the specific rights of every citizen' (Labour Party 1992b: 23) would surely lead, as would the similar intentions of the other parties in this area, to a body of law that was more specific about people's entitlements to personal social services and thereby a tighter, more enforceable, link between need and demand.

Two rather contradictory aspects define the Liberal Democrats' position on the future of the personal social services. On one hand, this is an area that is even more marginal to their central concerns than it is for the two other major parties. It received more scant mention in their 1992 manifesto than it did in those of Labour and the Tories. On the other hand, the Liberal Democrats appear to be alone amongst the three major parties in having explicitly addressed the issue of the right level of funding for the public personal social services. The reason for the low public priority given to this area by the Liberal Democrats is that they do not see it as a central concern to the voters that they wish to attract, predominantly younger electors more likely to be interested in the environment, constitutional reform and, amongst social policy issues, education. None the less, this low political salience of the issue in the party appears to have allowed those few within it who are concerned with the personal social services to adopt a more considered approach to the issues.

In particular, they have paid attention to the core problem of the needs–supply gap. In a substantial policy document published before the 1992 General Election it was pointed out that

> it is apparent that the present level of spending is not adequate to meet needs. The assumption behind the government proposals is that the only requirement is to provide alternatives to those presently entering residential care .... The fact is, there are an unidentified number of individuals living in the community with inadequate services, or no services at all, who also require assistance .... The Government's attempts to avoid this issue by making the provision of care entirely dependent on available resources means, in effect, that the most dependent will only receive services if they are taken away from others.
>
> (Liberal Democrats 1991e: 4.4.3–4)

The document then goes on to suggest that 'a Government

which is serious about care in the community is likely to be looking at an increase in spending of the order of one billion pounds per annum over a reasonably short period of time' (1991e: 4.4.5). One billion pounds is a rather large and round number and can only be taken to indicate a broad appreciation of the scale of the needs–supply gap that is at the heart of the policy problem presented by the personal social services. The published policy documents give no indication of how the bridging of the gap might be financed. One cannot but suspect that it is the unlikelihood of the Liberal Democratic party finding itself solely responsible for having to deal with the estimated shortfall that allowed it to give such a hostage – even if a minor one – to political fortune.

The Liberal Democrats' main declared policies for the personal social services are:

1 They would continue implementation of the impending major reforms brought about by the Community Care Act 1990, the Children Act 1989 and the Criminal Justice Act 1991.

2 They would introduce a charter of rights for people with disabilities and would implement sections 1–3 of the Disabled Persons Act 1986 which would provide an independent advocacy service.

3 They would ring-fence for up to three years money transferred from central to local government to pay for community care. They are opposed to long-term ring-fencing on the grounds that this would set ceilings rather than floors for expenditure. Many local authorities currently spend more than central government expects.

4 In addition to the compulsory assessment of all needy persons applying to the local authority, they would introduce separate assessment for carers.

5 Local authorities would receive bridging finance to assist them in introducing the new community care system.

6 They would in the longer term, as part of the reorganisation of local government, move to a system where both health and social services were the responsibility of the same level of local government.

7 The existing Invalid Care Allowance would be immediately increased by 15 per cent and made available to all those who

forgo normal earnings rather than just those under retirement age.

8 They would, in time, introduce 'individualised funding' for dependent people organised through a 'care brokerage' system. This is a radical idea, the product largely of experimentation in Canada (Laing 1991), which would mean that dependent people would not receive from the state very standardised sums of money like the Attendance Allowance and the Invalid Care Allowance but much more varied amounts depending upon their particular needs. In consultation with the brokerage service the money could be spent in a wide variety of ways, again depending on the person's particular needs and preferences.

9 They would set up an independent inspectorate of the social services and create a national General Social Services Council to oversee the provision of personal social services.

Again, it is likely that need and provision in this area would be more affected by the Liberal Democrats' wider policy intentions than by those changes specifically directed at the services. The party promised to increase the real value of the basic state pension (by £5 a week for a single person, £8 a week for a couple), to tie the pension to increases in average earnings and to make it payable independently of contribution records, thus reducing the need for many people to submit to Income Support means-tests. It is also the policy of the party to increase the real value of child benefit, to abolish the lower rate of Income Support for under-25s and to end cash-limiting of the Social Fund. All these changes are likely to reduce levels of financial need and increase people's ability to buy some of the services they require rather than turn to the social services. In the longer run the party has proposed to integrate the tax and benefit systems and to pay every adult in the population a basic benefit. A central plank of Liberal Democrat policy is the passing of a Bill of Rights and a Freedom of Information Act. Both of these would be likely to lead to test cases which seek to turn the largely discretionary services in this area into absolute social rights.

To conclude: the Labour Party is almost as careful as the Conservatives to avoid commitments that might substantially increase expenditure on the personal social services. Only the

Liberal Democrats have spoken, rather loosely, of spending more. It is impossible to predict from any existing policy positions specific effects on the nature and amount of the services. There is an understandable, rational and historically-based failure in any of the available policy literature to engage with the core problem of how the volume of resources in this area is to be determined. It is not in the interests of a party electorally, or in terms of its potential future as a government, to recognise the huge needs–supply gap. It is likely that a Labour or a Liberal Democrat government, or some coalition of the two, would expand provision for the personal social services only in those cases where short-term political expediency made it unavoidable, for example in response to public outcry about some discovery of ill-treatment, or where some policy reform accidentally allowed the huge volume of pent-up need to be turned into effective demand.

DEMAND FOR PERSONAL SOCIAL SERVICES IN THE 1990s

In his 1970 essay on 'The future of the personal social services' Roy Parker observes that 'in the past the quality, extent and nature of the personal social services have been largely supply-determined' and goes on to consider the possibility that in the future 'real needs may find more forceful expression in effective demands' (Parker 1970: 109). Amongst the possible sources of additional demand for local social services he surveyed were: more dependent elderly, more children, more children with disabilities surviving into adulthood, greater geographical mobility, the special problems of a growing number of ethnic minority families, the needs of more working mothers with young children, more families coping with the care of members who in an earlier age would have received permanent institutional care, the deleterious effects of poorly built environments on mutual aid systems, the decline in the number of older, single women in the population who, traditionally, have performed much care work, more information about needs and the shortcomings of services, increased power of professional groups to demand more and better services, and greater consumer participation in service policies. It is remarkable, but on consideration perhaps not very surprising, how well this list summarises the possibilities of increased demand today.

It has been argued so far that expenditure on the local authority social services has tended to grow faster than overall public expenditure largely because of the tendency over time for more and more of the suppressed and pent-up need to escape and to express itself as effective demand. It is likely that this pattern will continue in the future despite the government's efforts to establish a more explicitly rationed service. Indeed, the very radical nature of the recent changes itself is likely to be a source of additional demand. As has been argued, major reforms tend to shift the personal social services upwards to new levels of expenditure even when that was not the basic intention. The remainder of this chapter considers possible sources of increased demand during the 1990s.

Perhaps the most important source of new effective demand will result from the central place that has been given to individual assessment of need within the new community care arrangements. Assessment is to be a distinct part of the process of arranging care. 'The Government proposes that the responsibility for ensuring that an assessment is made should be a specific duty of the local authority' (Departments of Health, Social Security, Wales and Scotland 1989: para 3.2.7). This will be done 'in collaboration with medical, nursing and other interests . . . assessing individual need, designing care arrangements and securing their delivery within available resources' (1989: para 1.12). It is clear that the intention of assessment is not to expand demand but rather to meet it in the most cost-effective manner possible and particularly to 'avoid unnecessary institutional care by ensuring that decisions on the provision of services are made on the basis of a careful assessment of need' (1989: para 2.12).

However, many local authorities are very concerned as to the volume of resources that the whole assessment process will absorb. First, it is becoming clear that assessment will be almost a social entitlement for a whole range of people, many of whom in the past were unlikely to have come into contact with the social services at all. 'Local authorities should ensure that means of referral are widely publicised. They should also establish, and make public, criteria of eligibility for assessment, and the way in which their assessment processes will work' (1989: para 3.2.9). Although the legislation gives the local authorities discretion as to the criteria which will entitle people to an assessment in the first place it is clear it will not be possible to make this unduly restrictive. In particular, assessments will have to be made before many old people can leave hospital and go into a residential or nursing home.

Second, Department of Health guidance is requiring that the assessments will often be done in collaboration with GPs and other relevant care professionals in the health, education and housing services. The local authorities are required to take the lead in co-ordinating these joint assessments and doubtless this will be very time consuming. Third, the Department of Health is also insisting that the assessment be needs-based and not merely consider whether an individual would benefit from existing and available services. All in all, it is difficult to see how the whole assessment process can be prevented from becoming both very costly to carry out and a basis from which needy people and their supporters can demand services or highlight deficiencies. There is a distinct possibility that this mechanism, originally conceived of as a more accurate rationing device, will come to be seen as a social right and a passport to other services. Unfulfilled assessment will become a prime weapon for criticising the performance of the social services. The two opposition parties have even talked of a separate right to assessment for informal carers.

The 1989 White Paper recognised that 'people from different cultural backgrounds may have particular care needs and problems' and that if the assessments are carried out as intended they will certainly be a source of extra demand for services more attuned to the needs of cultural minorities. Hitherto the social services have found it difficult to respond appropriately to the requirements of minorities and they are particularly ill-prepared to deal with what will rapidly become a large group of potential users, elderly people who grew up in a different culture (Glendenning and Pearson 1988; Norman 1986; Prime 1987).

The failure of the welfare state generally to grasp the implications of an increasingly multi-cultural society is just one example of a more general reason why the personal social services may continue to grow faster than other parts of the welfare system. They have always been a service of last resort. It is likely that in the future social services departments will be increasingly vulnerable to demands deflected from other parts of the welfare system, particularly from the health services. Most important amongst these is the continuing decline in the number of geriatric beds in National Health hospitals and the central part that short bed-stays play in the search for efficiency gains. Until recently it was possible for hospitals to move old people directly to private nursing homes with the costs met from social security. From April 1993 this will only be possible after a social service assessment and if the relevant local authority has the funds necessary to pay for the care element of institutional care. Social services are likely to come under considerable pressure from hospitals to act quickly.

More threatening to demand than the hospital sector's declining capacity for care, as distinct from treatment, is the possibility of a decline in the caring role of the family. The family is the core institution that protects the formal personal social services from overwhelming demand. However, it is not certain that traditional social definitions of family obligation and particularly of women's obligations to care will be sustained in the future. The divorce rate in Britain is one of the highest in the world: four out of ten marriages now fail (Haskey 1988). One child in four now lives in a reconstituted family or with a lone parent (Kiernan and Wicks 1990). It is not clear that these children will feel the same obligations to care for their elderly parents, or that their parents will expect it.

The role of the family in the care of the dependant is complicated, varied and ambiguous. Traditional assumptions and practices remain strong and important (Finch and Mason 1990). Family care continues to be by far the most important form of social care for old people. On the other hand, public policy makers need to be very careful about relying on these institutions. Family practices are much more varied than they used to be. The values of kinship obligation have to compete with others to do with work and independence. Patterns of household formation are similarly more varied and the consequent arrangements more fragile and to that extent less reliable. Public policy about caring must operate in much more varied and uncertain territory. Yet none of the major parties proposed even the beginnings of a family policy in their 1992 manifestos. Little account is taken in current personal social service policies of the substantial changes in family organisation and structure that lie behind relatively modest changes in broad demographic numbers.

Over time, the 'failures' of both the public and private care systems tend to find their way into social service budgets even if the routes are rather long and indirect and have little to do with distinct or planned party policies. Two related examples are illustrative:

first, the perennial waves of concern about child welfare, and second, the chronic tendency of governments to establish special, protected budgets to deal with high profile social problems.

The standard spending assessments for local authorities in 1992–3 include an increase in funding for training from £7 million to £29 million (DoH and OPCS 1992). This is largely a consequence of public concern and media attention, not necessarily the same thing, about recent failures in child protection, in particular concern about the scale of child sexual abuse and, more recently, about unsatisfactory regimes in children's homes. Indeed, we can see here the beginnings of another cycle of what has become almost the classic post-war route to expansion in effective demand for more and better social work. Described very summarily, but without severe damage to the truth, it can be said that it was the death in 1944 of a young boy, Denis O'Neill, through ill-treatment in foster care, that led through committees of inquiry to the Children Act of 1948 and the establishment of a professional child care service (Packman 1975: 5–18). Later, when in the 1960s public concern turned to the growth of 'juvenile delinquency', this new profession was able to support another round of committees in their successful pressure for further legislation (the 1969 Children and Young Persons Act) which led directly to the substantial expansion of the personal social services in the 1970s (1975: 103–29). Now in the late 1980s and early 1990s the process has begun again. Following another spate of rare media attention on personal social service issues, the Butler-Sloss report on responses to discoveries of child abuse and the Kahan, Utting and Warner reports on child care in residential institutions have all recommended more specialist training and further professionalisation. There is little doubt that the eventual result will be an expanded public service and a more effective professional lobby for another dimension of the personal social services.

As has already been mentioned, one of the few areas of difference between the political parties in the run-up to the 1992 General Election was whether part of central government's grant to local authorities should be 'ring-fenced' to pay for community care. In fact a practice of isolating parts of both revenue and capital expenditure is well established. In addition to the specific training grant, in 1992–3 local authorities received specific grants covering services for people with AIDS/HIV, the provision of community care services for the mentally ill, the provision of services for drug and alcohol misusers and the development of the guardian *ad litem* services required by the Children Act (DoH and OPCS 1992: 21). All of these are areas of public and media attention and are potentially high growth areas of social service expenditure. They are also examples of problems which cannot be adequately absorbed by the informal sector, the family, but which are rather reflections or consequences of changes in the nature and organisation of the family.

Richard Titmuss once remarked that 'whenever the British people have identified and investigated a social problem there has followed a national call for more social work and more trained social workers' (Titmuss 1968: 85). Policy developments in the personal social services are almost always reactive and spasmodic. Titmuss was referring to one stage of the cycle of policy development in which governments are forced to react and pay the price of an expanded service. This is almost always followed by a second stage in which the politicians attempt to reassert control and set rules and establish ways of rationing resources. These are soon upset by a fresh set of social issues which must be responded to. The end of the 1980s, by coincidence, marked a point at which much legislation in the two principal areas of social service activity, child protection and community care, had sought to re-establish control over this largely reactive area of social expenditure. If the lessons of history are reliable it will soon be undermined by unexpected social issues and the need for short-term responses. The logic of this cycle is unlikely to be much affected by whichever of the major parties is in charge of central government at the time, or even by the severe constraints on public expenditure that are likely to dominate the period up to and around the turn of the century.

Chapter 9

Housing
Need, equity, ownership and the economy

Clare Ungerson

In considering the politics of housing policy, there are a number of ways – or discourses – which can be used to understand and analyse the dimensions of these politics. These discourses are, first, the question of 'housing need' – how need is determined through political and economic processes, and which policies will best satisfy defined 'needs'; second, the question of housing equity – how best to ensure that households on similar incomes receive similar levels of state assistance with their housing costs, and that there is a linear relationship between payment on the one hand and the quality and quantity of housing on the other; third, the question of housing ownership – the economic and social relations between owners and their tenants, and the desirability, or otherwise, of developing particular forms of tenure; and fourth, the question of the interdependent relationship between the management of housing policy and the management of the economy as a whole, and how far investment in housing, particularly new construction, can and should be used as an economic regulator.

This chapter is written largely within the framework of the first discourse – namely, the politics of housing need and the way in which the different political parties proposed, at the time of the April 1992 General Election, to define 'need' and to satisfy it. However, it would be misleading to suggest that the politics of need were the only, indeed an important, element of the discourse at the time: rather more important, certainly as far as the Conservative Party was concerned, was the discourse of ownership, while the discourse of equity, particularly as far as the Liberal Democrat Party was concerned, was just as important as the question of need.

But it is equally noticeable that the whole question of housing policy received relatively little attention in any of the three manifestos: of far more importance was the question of economic management as a whole, and other social policy areas such as health and education. However, as far as housing policy is concerned, over the period during which this chapter was being written – from March to October 1992 – the dominant discourse changed, and, in terms of general politics, housing policy became very important. In the aftermath of the General Election, it became clear that the economic recession was growing, if anything, deeper and more firmly embedded. This had two effects on the politics of housing policy. First, the fourth discourse – that of the relationship of housing policy, and particularly policies for new house construction, to economic management as a whole – shifted firmly into view. This was not a new idea, and clearly arose out of the Keynesian traditions of both Labour and Liberal Democrat Parties. In their manifestos, as we shall see, both these parties had advocated the promotion of new housing construction as a stimulus to economic growth. But the second way in which the discourse shifted is that the relationship between what happens in one segment of the housing system – namely, owner occupation – and what happens in the rest of the economy also came to the fore. During the few months after the election, it was increasingly and very publicly argued that it was the rate of failure of households to maintain mortgage payments in the owner-occupied sector that was feeding a slow but steady drop in house prices and a general flatness in consumer confidence and hence in consumer demand, and that this constituted a major reason for the inability of the British economy to climb out of recession. In the short term, political arguments developed as to how best to break the crisis in the owner-occupied market – whether through increasing tax breaks for all, or for those on low income only, or by generating schemes whereby owners in trouble could become, partially and temporarily, tenants. In the long term, political arguments began to develop around the whole area of the third discourse I have identified – namely, how far expansion in the tenure of owner occupation should be allowed to go, and to what extent, and how, renting should be revived within either the privately rented or the publicly rented sector, or some hybrid of the two.

But before turning to a more detailed discussion of these political differences, it is important to understand their historical context. Thus the following section discusses briefly the way in which the housing policies of the 1980s shifted the burden of costs for housing provision from state to consumer, as well as the main aspects of the 'housing problem' as it emerged at the end of that decade.

FROM STATE TO CONSUMER – SQUARING HOUSING CIRCLES IN THE 1980s

In a White Paper on housing policy published in September 1987, the Conservative government spelled out its objectives, of which there were four: to revive the privately rented sector; to give council tenants the right to transfer to other landlords; to target public subsidy on those households with the worst problems; and to continue to encourage the growth of home ownership (DoE 1987a). However, a historian writing in the twenty-first century will almost certainly place the extension of owner occupation as the first rather than the fourth aim of government in the 1980s. The route to this strategic aim, in a market situation and uniquely malleable to government, was the sale of its own property – council houses and flats – to sitting tenants. But this tactic to fulfil the first aim was also part and parcel of the second strategic aim, namely to reduce the local authority sector of the housing system, such that this tenure was likely either to disappear altogether or to become a tiny rump providing only for the statutorily homeless. To this end, central government grant to local housing authorities was drastically reduced and instead some – largely rhetorical rather than practical – emphasis was placed on the development of housing associations as providers of rented housing and purchasers of existing council housing. A new name for housing allocated not entirely by the price mechanism was coined: 'social housing'. A mixture of local authority, housing association and co-operative owners, this sector was expected to house those still unable to move into owner occupation, and to house them at – another new term – 'affordable' (but closer to market) rents. This rents policy was in turn part of the third strategic aim, which was to introduce the market into previously non-market parts of the housing system. Rents of council houses had, by the end of the decade, to reflect a reasonable return on the capital values of the dwellings themselves; somewhat similarly, housing associations were forced to increase the amount of capital raised from private sources, and then increase their rents in order to draw close to covering market-related historic costs, if not market rents. The fourth strategic aim was to increase the provision of rented housing, not in the public sector but in the privately rented sector, partially by deregulation of rents and relaxation of security of tenure particularly for new tenancies, but also by providing considerable producer subsidy, through the Business Expansion Scheme, in the form of tax breaks for those willing to invest, on a temporary basis, in accommodation new to the privately rented sector and let at market rents.

Thus it was generally expected that households would themselves increasingly bear the 'true' costs of their housing consumption within a largely private and increasingly marketised system. Nevertheless, it was also accepted that some households in the rented sector would need some maintenance of their effective demand particularly to generate increased supply in the privately rented sector. This was to be guaranteed under the Housing Benefit system reorganised within the ambit of the 1986 social security reforms. But Housing Benefit was also, of course, available in the publicly rented sector. Indeed, the increasing use of Housing Benefit, particularly in the public sector, could be said to have been a fifth strategic aim of housing policy insofar as it was a part of the general aim of government to 'target' all benefits on those demonstrably in 'need' rather than provide general and sometimes universal subsidy. The shift from 'producer' subsidies to 'consumer' subsidies in the public housing sector was a very important part of the overarching policy for selectivity and targeting in social security policy which spilled over – literally – into the housing system.

Like many other aspects of Thatcherite social policy, these housing policies amounted to radical and pervasive change. Moreover, the implementation of most of them was, within the terms of the policies themselves, a considerable success. The proportion of the housing stock in owner occupation expanded from 55.8 per cent in 1981 to 67.6 per cent in 1991 (see Table 9.1). As a result of the 'right to buy' given to sitting council tenants in 1980, local authorities and new towns sold almost 1.5 million homes during the 1980s (CSO 1992a: 147). Rents for local authority properties rose steadily, and, from the mid-1980s onwards, increasingly faster than the rate of inflation (CSO 1992a: 152). Similarly, as a result of the implementation of the 1988 Housing Act introducing

Table 9.1 Stock of dwellings by tenure. Nations of the UK, 1981–91 (per cent)

	Owner occupied		Rented from private owners and other tenures		Rented from housing associations		Rented from local authorities or new town corporations	
	April 1981	December 1991	April 1981	December 1991	April 1981	December 1991	April 1981	December 1991
England	57.7	69.1	11.4	7.6	2.3	3.2	28.6	20.1
Wales	61.8	72.0	9.7	6.6	1.0	2.5	27.5	18.9
Scotland	35.6	52.8	10.1	5.5	1.7	3.3	52.6	38.4
Northern Ireland	53.1	65.6	7.8	3.5	0.4	2.0	38.6	28.5
UK	**55.8**	**67.6**	**11.2**	**7.3**	**2.1**	**3.1**	**31.0**	**21.9**

Source: DoE 1992: Table 9.4

a new market-orientated financial regime for housing associations, rents in that sector had risen by just over 60 per cent over two years by the end of 1990 (IBH 1991). Local authorities had practically ceased to be providers of new housing: the number of new council dwellings built dropped from 86,000 in 1980 to 13,000 in 1991.

By the end of the 1980s council housing was no longer a constituent of demand on the public purse, but a provider of public monies. According to the Joseph Rowntree Foundation the proceeds from council house sales between 1987/8 and 1989/90 amounted to £33 billion (1990/1 prices), which was 'more than the proceeds from privatising BP, British Telecom, British Airways, Rolls-Royce and British Gas all put together' (IBH 1991: 70). Central government restricted local authority expenditure of such capital receipts on housing at first to 20 per cent of the proceeds in any one year, and later, as part of the Local Government and Housing Act 1989, to 25 per cent; moreover, after 1989 local authorities had to spend the remaining 75 per cent on redeeming their general debts. Niner and Maclennan suggest that by 1989 local housing authorities unable to spend their capital receipts had accumulated £8 billion of 'enforced savings'. This in turn generated interest which substantially fed into current Housing Revenue Accounts to the tune of covering 10 per cent of current housing expenditure (Niner and Maclennan 1990: 50). Indeed, some local authorities found themselves so flush with money on Housing Revenue Account that they were able to use the surplus to transfer many millions into their general rate funds (Malpass 1990: 152). In the 1980s, rental income for public housing moved from a less than 50 per cent contribution to far and away the most important contributor to Housing Revenue Account, outstripping central government housing subsidy, rate fund contribution and interest on capital receipts put together, by a ratio of more than 2 to 1 by 1986/7 (Hills and Mullings 1990: 150–4).

The political ease with which this particular version of 'squaring the circle' was accomplished was generated by the expansion of heavily targeted housing benefit coupled with the 'right to buy'. Between 1985/6 and 1990/1 aggregate expenditure on housing benefit increased from £4.5 billion to £5.3 billion (IBH 1991: 20). However, throughout the 1980s housing benefit tapers were steadily increased for those households on incomes above Supplementary Benefit levels culminating in the 1988 changes to the social security system which put in place a 65 per cent taper on net income (Hills and Mullings 1990: 191–4); in 1983 households on 110 per cent of average male gross earnings had been eligible for Housing Benefit, but by April 1988, only households on less than 50 per cent of average male gross earnings were able to claim (IBH 1991: 20). This in itself has constituted a powerful incentive for those tenants not eligible for Housing Benefit, but facing very large rent increases, to seek to enter owner occupation either through exercising their 'right to buy' or by moving into the conventional market. Not surprisingly the numbers of households claiming the benefit decreased (CSO 1992a: 154). But for many of those households lucky enough to stay in the system (largely because they were pensioners or unemployed), and who were tenants in the public sector, their rent was automatically covered to the tune of 100 per cent, including any rent increase. For this group then, housing in effect became free at the point of consumption – a situation about which they were clearly not going to protest.

However, there was one area of housing policy which remained apparently impervious to the new broom of market ideology and which grew in importance in political terms. This was the largest consumer subsidy of them all: mortgage interest tax relief (MITR). This outstripped expenditure on Housing Benefit for the first time in 1980/1 and, in aggregate, has moved further and further away from transfer payments to tenants ever since (IBH 1991: 17). The Conservative government occasionally tried to control this expenditure, in particular capping it at £30,000 in 1983, but increases in owner occupation, in the price of housing, and in the number of mortgages reaching the £30,000 limit, meant that the actual aggregate tax expenditure on MITR continued to climb inexorably between 1981/2 and 1990/1 from £3.9 billion to £7.7 billion (1990/1 prices) (CSO 1992a: 156).

MAKING ENDS MEET: INCOMES, COSTS AND NEEDS

Thus there was during the 1980s, with the single exception of the Business Expansion Scheme for the privately rented sector, a radical shift away from producer subsidies towards 'market prices' combined with consumer subsidies. The impact on households was considerable. In the public sector, those tenants not able to claim their full rent through Housing Benefit were increasingly only able to 'square their own circle' either through shifting into owner occupation or through running up rent arrears. Between 1979 and 1990 the average proportion of rent collectable that was in arrears rose from 3.2 per cent to 8.2 per cent in England and Wales. Arrears in some London boroughs, where rents were particularly high, had reached astonishing proportions (up to 90 per cent in one borough) (Bucknall 1991). A similar phenomenon began to appear in the owner-occupied sector: a huge leap in average mortgage outgoings as a percentage of net income took place in 1989 and 1990, reaching 40.5 per cent of net income in 1990 (IBH 1991: 15). While this partially reflected two short-run trends – the exceptionally rapid rise in house prices in 1988 and 1989 (IBH 1991: 35) and the exceptionally high real mortgage interest rates which very sharply increased over the period 1988–90 (CSO 1992a: 152) – the steady increase in mortgage outgoings as a proportion of net income that has occurred since 1970 also reflects the long-run trend of the entry into this tenure of lower-income households. It is not surprising that the incidence of mortgage arrears steadily increased during the 1980s. In 1981, there were 21,500 households in arrears by six to twelve months' payments, but by 1991 this had increased eightfold to 162,200 households, plus there were a further 59,700 households in arrears of over twelve months (CSO 1992a: 154). In July 1992 the Council of Mortgage Lenders announced that over 300,000 households were then in arrears of at least six months (*Independent*, 30 July 1992). Inevitably, building societies had taken action on many of these cases; in 1990, 107,000 warrants for repossession of residential property were issued, and 42,000 were executed (CSO 1992a: 154). Both the government in 1991 and building societies in 1992 attempted, through a variety of 'mortgage to rent' schemes for owners in trouble, to stem the haemorrhage of foreclosed properties on to an already stagnant market but these schemes, particularly that sponsored by the government, met with very limited success.

Rent and mortgage arrears became an increasingly important reason reported by those households *accepted* as 'homeless' as the precipitating reason for their predicament (CSO 1992a: 150). However, many authorities treated arrears, whether of mortgage or rent, as the equivalent of 'intentional homelessness', thus avoiding responsibility for re-accommodating even those households falling into the fairly narrowly defined 'priority need' category under the homelessness legislation (Widdowson 1987). The effective demand of these households, eroded by rising interest rates and rising rents, and unprotected by legal rights to housing, meant that annually many thousands of households failed to thrive, and disappeared altogether. Similarly, the withdrawal of Income Support from 16–17-year-olds not participating in a Youth Training Scheme completely abolished the effective demand of a particular demographic and social group, and led to an apparent explosion of homelessness among young people. Household fission became an increasingly anxious and difficult process, while household fusion, through loss of effective demand, became the increasingly likely lot of many hundreds of thousands of households.

While many of these processes of fission and fusion were relatively invisible, unaccounted for and unaccountable, certain kinds of homelessness were increasingly discussed in the media and increasingly visible on the streets. Ragged encampments of roofless individuals appeared in the very heart of tourist, legal and media London and in many other cities. While these homeless individuals were obviously the detritus of households which had failed to thrive, they constituted a tiny minority of the general mass of homeless households. But this rising tide of 'homeless' applicants, successful and otherwise, was no adequate indicator of general housing 'need'. For example, single people, unless accompanied by children or defined as 'vulnerable' through age or disability, had no rights for rehousing under the homelessness legislation. Both applicants and acceptances were the end products of a long process of personal and political definition, legitimation, formation, and 'acceptable' failure.

Housing 'need' has both highly visible and highly invisible elements to it. Rotting and obsolete slums; massive tower blocks, unsuitable for the housing of children but nevertheless full of single-parent families, covered in graffiti and scarred with concrete cancer; whole families eating, sleeping and living in one room in rundown 'hotels'; people sleeping 'rough': all these are the relatively visible aspects of housing 'need'. But paradoxically, the other elements of misery and anxiety induced by, for example, rents and mortgages no longer falling within the family budget; the difficulty of forming separate households, not just for people of all ages trapped in violent and abusive families but also for young people reaching an age where the cultural expectation is that they should be able to leave the parental home; old people desperate to remain in their own homes, but no longer able to maintain them properly: these are some of the relatively invisible aspects of housing 'need' which deeply affect the lives and relationships of millions.

PARADOX, PARALYSIS AND NEEDS IN THE 1990s

Despite these complexities of defining need in housing, it is nevertheless possible to see that during a recession such as Britain experienced in the late 1980s and early 1990s, even for well-established and culturally legitimated households, household formation and maintenance became a frustrating and frightening experience such that the concept of 'need' appears to have simplified. For a great many individual households in the majority tenure of owner occupation there was, as we have seen, a major problem for their personal finances. But even more worrying was that for those trying to extricate themselves from a mortgage that was now costing more than they could afford, the exit route was blocked – in two ways. First, the drop in house prices both reflected and created a seizing-up of housing transactions: estate agents in the early 1990s continuously reported an unprece-dented lack of potential buyers. Second, many mortgagors, estimated by some experts to be as many as 1.5 million (*Independent*, 30 July 1992), found that their mortgage was actually more than the declining value of their house; even if they did exit from owner occupation and manage to sell their house, they would still be in debt but without the benefit of occupying the original source of their indebtedness. At the same time the market was increasingly glutted with houses put on the market by the building societies anxious to get the benefit of foreclosure and repossession.

Thus the market for owner occupation was apparently paralysed and dangerously close to free fall, while many households were trapped in a deep pit at the bottom. But it was even worse than this: at risk too was the safety of the national domestic economy. By the end of the 1980s it had been realised that the owner-occupied housing market had a very considerable effect on consumer spending and thus on the economy as a whole. During the period of house price increases between 1988 and 1989, mortgagors, with full agreement of the by now deregulated lending agencies, had been able to bolster their spending capacity very considerably by using the security of their increasingly valuable property to finance further loans and expenditure. This so-called 'equity withdrawal' has been estimated to amount to as much as £25–30 billion in 1988 alone. By 1989 all the important models of the UK economy had incorporated assumptions about the positive impact of increases in house prices on consumer spending (Pearce and Wilcox 1991: 33–4). One has therefore to assume that in a period of house price *decreases*, there are bound to be concomitant effects *downwards* on consumer spending. Thus in a recession, efforts to increase consumer spending in order to boost the economy generally through, for example, fiscal policy, can be stymied by the prevailing circumstances of the owner-occupied housing market. As more and more households on the margins of financial viability have been drawn into owner occupation, so the risks of these households faltering under changing circumstances and bringing the housing market down with them have increased. Similarly, as owner occupation has grown into the major houser of the British people, so its tentacles have spread into all economic activity. Increasingly, the tail wags the dog: a booming housing market entails a booming and probably overheating economy, while a static and depressed housing market entails a depressed economy. Moreover, a vicious circle ensues, since a faltering housing market leads to major problems in the construction industry – in 1991/2 house completions fell by 10 per cent (CEEFAX, 4 August 1992) – which, in a labour-intensive industry, leads to serious increases in unemployment.

Thus it is no longer just a question of how to square the circle within the relatively narrow area of housing policy, but rather how to stop the housing system from flooding the arena. However, quite apart from these macro-problems of the management of the British economy arising out of change and paralysis in the housing market, it was also clear by the end of the 1980s that there was another direct threat to enterprise on a micro and personal basis. As a consequence of the emphasis that the Conservative government had placed on targeting the 'needy', the entire system of transfer payments had become more and more entrapping. Nowhere is this more obvious than for low-income households claiming Housing Benefit where a marginal 'tax' rate prevailed of 87 pence in the pound (Pearce and Wilcox 1991: 30–1). But even worse than this 'poverty trap' is the 'unemployment trap'. Here, it is frequently much better for individuals and households to remain unemployed and dependent on Income Support than to move into paid work. This is particularly true of owner occupiers. As soon as they move off Income Support into paid work, they lose all financial support for their mortgage, except for MITR, which at low income is of least benefit to them (Pearce and Wilcox 1991: 29). Thus, para-doxically, by trying to encourage self-help and independence and at the same time reduce public expenditure, the level and permanence of dependency on state benefit for nearly two million households has been deepened.

WHAT IS TO BE DONE? THE CONSERVATIVE VIEW

For the moment, Majorism, at least as far as housing policy is concerned, seems little different from Thatcherism. John Major has stressed not only the continuity he feels with important aspects of his predecessor's policy but, if anything, he has opted to stress even further one particular aspect of it. Significantly, the title of his 'Selected speeches during his first year as Prime Minister' is *The Power to Choose: The Right to Own* (Major 1991). John Major has placed ownership of all kinds at the centre of his philosophy, as is evident from his speech to the Conservative Party Conference at Blackpool in October 1991:

> In the 1980s we began a great revolution. Our aim was a life enriched by ownership, in which homes, shares and pensions were not something for others, but something for everyone. . . . But this revolution is still not complete. In the 1990s we must carry it further. We must extend savings and ownership in every form. We now have the chance to make enduring change. For people in their middle years are inheriting homes, businesses and farms on a scale never before seen. The pioneers of the property-owning democracy are the parents of the capital-owning democracy to come. . . . I want to see wealth cascading down the generations.

Thus the Conservatives were still moving strongly in the direction of the expansion of owner occupation. This was confirmed by the 1992 election manifesto, which echoed Major's words and stated that:

> The opportunity to own a home and pass it on is one of the

most important rights an individual has in a free society. Conservatives have extended that right. It lies at the heart of our philosophy.

(Conservative Party 1992: 33)

To that end, the manifesto promised to 'maintain mortgage tax relief' (though it did not specify at what rate), continue the 'right to buy', introduce a 'rents to mortgages' scheme for council tenants (a promise fulfilled in July 1992), and put more of the Housing Corporation's existing budget into equity share home ownership schemes. Thus the Conservative manifesto was very predominantly written within the third discourse of housing politics identified earlier – namely that of the politics of property ownership and tenure.

However, despite the fact that Major stresses again and again the desirability of home ownership, there was recognition both in the manifesto and in practice that some kind of rented sector had to be maintained. This first came to public notice when, largely because of the total stagnation in the market for owner occupation, and also possibly because of the political sensitivity of the issue and the proximity of a general election, the new Major government introduced an emergency 'mortgage to rent' scheme for owner occupiers threatened with repossession because of mortgage arrears. It is arguable, particularly since stamp duty on house purchase was temporarily suspended at the same time, that this was a policy to stop the rot in owner occupation rather than to promote renting. However, there are other signs that some re-emphasis is returning to renting, particularly in the 'social renting' sector. Here the manifesto reiterated the promise, made first in 1991, to push £6 billion into the Housing Corporation to 'provide' 153,000 homes over three years from 1992 onwards. This will be a very considerable upturn in new provision by housing associations; a rate of 50,000 new housing association dwellings per year for the next three years compares extremely favourably with the years 1988–90 where the annual average increase in housing association dwellings was 15,000 (CSO 1992a: 146). The manifesto also mentioned that 'we are determined to encourage a strong private rented sector while continuing to safeguard the rights of existing regulated tenants' (Conservative Party 1992: 33); but the means to this objective are weak, amounting to enabling home owners to 'rent a room', free of tax on the rental income. In the light of the 1992 budget's announced intention to bring all Business Expansion Scheme tax breaks to an end in 1993 – which will particularly affect the generous producer subsidy to private landlords – this very much smaller producer subsidy seems feeble indeed. Finally, the future of housing policy, at least as far as the old-style 'council housing' is concerned, looks certain. If recent policies continue, council housing will become a method through which government collects revenue rather than spends it.

Thus the 1992 Conservative manifesto, as far as housing policy is concerned, was indeed a very conservative document. The policies of the 1980s, and most particularly of the 1988 Housing Act, are to stay in place and be enacted into the 1990s. A slight shift in emphasis towards 'social housing' let at 'affordable' rents (but nevertheless close to historic costs) is detectable, possibly in deference to public concern about increasing – and increasingly visible – homelessness. But the major issues of difficulties of access to owner occupation for low-income households combined with the problems such households have in shouldering their commitments to high and variable mortgages once they are in the tenure, lack of Income Support for 16- and 17-year-olds, of decreasing hostel provision for homeless people, of the particular housing problems that single people are increasingly experiencing – all these were left unmentioned and untouched. A foreigner reading this manifesto might think that Britain's housing problems in 1992 were largely confined to the question of who owns property; and then, in the middle of tourist London, be struck by the hundreds of homeless people openly living on the streets and camping in the verdant public squares.

PUSHING THE ALTERNATIVE: LIBERAL DEMOCRAT AND LABOUR

Not surprisingly, both the major opposition parties couched much of their discussion of housing policy within the discourses of 'need', economic management and equity. The Labour Party began its manifesto with a pastiche poem by Adrian Henri entitled *Winter Ending*; this considers the way in which a Labour victory would impact need, and on housing in particular:

> As the last cardboard boxes
> are swept away beneath busy bridges,
> the cold blue landscape of winter
> suddenly alive with bright red roses.

But the mention of 'cardboard boxes' is the nearest Labour came in the manifesto to cataloguing housing need. In contrast, the Liberal Democrats, in the first chapter of their manifesto entitled 'Britain's balance sheet', drew attention to the drop in council house building, the increase in homelessness acceptances, and in mortgage arrears (Liberal Democrats 1992: 17). But both manifestos, particularly the Labour one, stressed the centrality of housing investment as part of a programme of economic recovery. In Labour's first chapter, entitled 'Immediate action for national recovery', under the sub-heading 'Action for industry', the following paragraph appeared:

> We will immediately begin the phased release of receipts from the sale of council houses, land and property receipts to allow local authorities to build new homes and improve old ones. More building workers in the recession-savaged construction and building supply industries will be employed and more families rehoused. Equivalent arrangements will be made in Scotland.
>
> (Labour Party 1992b: 10)

In a similar chapter entitled 'Britain's prosperity: public investment; private enterprise' the Liberal Democrats, in a rather less specific statement, said they would 'attack unemployment' by increasing spending on 'public transport, housing, hospitals and schools' (Liberal Democrats 1992: 20).

But it is also interesting to note that neither party went so far as to *quantify* need, produce figures to indicate *how much* public investment would be made in house construction, or produce *targets* for annual housing starts and completions. This is in stark contrast to the competitive target setting that prevailed when the needs discourse predominated in housing politics during the 1950s and 1960s. In somewhat confessional mood the Labour Party had, in their policy document for housing published the previous year, made it clear that they eschewed target setting for housing:

> It is not desirable to fix a single, simple national target figure

for the number of new homes to be built or improved each year. Indeed, the adoption of simplistic targets in the past led to a fixation with quantity at the expense of quality. Too many people are living with the planning mistakes of the fifties and sixties. We have no plans to return to the system built estates of that era.

(Labour Party 1991d: 17)

It is of course possible to have targets without, at the same time, becoming obsessed with quantity or committed to system-built housing. A report published by the Audit Commission shortly after the election did produce targets, but, as that report made clear, such numbers are based on assumptions about household formation and effective demand which are difficult to predict, and subject to the impacts of policies of rights to housing, particularly of single people, and of income maintenance (Audit Commission 1992: 6–7, and Appendix 1). It is perhaps symptomatic of a Labour Party committed to caution that it felt unable to tackle these kinds of political considerations head on. However, both Labour and the Liberal Democrats did have policies designed to deal with the needs they *did* identify, and in these they were strikingly similar. They were agreed that provision for the homeless was seriously deficient and both had similar proposals to bring empty property, owned by both public and private landlords, into immediate use to ease the problem of the long-term placement of homeless people in bed and breakfast hotels. Both parties also clearly recognised that there is a problem of effective demand, both in terms of income and of rights to housing for some particular groups. For example, both Labour and Liberal Democrats proposed to reinstate Income Support for 16- and 17-year-olds, and to bring to an end the lower rate of Income Support for those under 25; the Liberal Democrats also proposed to reinstate housing benefit for students and to make Family Credit reflect mortgage interest payments, thus ameliorating the unemployment trap for mortgagors. Neither party proposed to do away with Housing Benefit altogether although both had proposals that would have reduced the sharpness of the taper. Finally, the Labour Party in its strategy document proposed that the definition of 'priority need' for action under the homelessness legislation be widened until eventually there would be no exclusions, but that immediately the category should be widened to include single people.

However, it was within the 'equity' discourse that the opposition parties developed their main differences. In 1989, the then Social and Liberal Democrats had published an 'English White Paper' entitled *Housing: a Time for Action*. This outlined a new regime for the whole of housing finance and proposed, among many other changes, to abolish MITR and use the large sums saved thereby to promote a new form of rented housing, subsidised through both substantial producer and consumer subsidies and called 'Partnership Housing'. This proposal found its way into the Liberal Democrat manifesto, where it was stated that:

> We will encourage home ownership, but we recognise that the housing market has been distorted by mortgage tax relief, and we believe that choice in housing means providing more rented accommodation in both public and private sectors. We will: *Introduce housing cost relief* weighted towards those most in need and available to house buyers *and* renters. This will replace mortgage tax relief for future home buyers, which often helps most those who need it least, and causes enormous distortions in the savings and housing markets.
>
> (Liberal Democrats 1992: 36)

In contrast the Labour Party, perhaps because it had a more realistic chance of being elected, played much safer and committed itself to the maintenance of MITR at 'the present rate' (Labour Party 1992b: 20). This appeared to be somewhat enigmatically hinting that MITR be allowed to wither on the vine so that eventual abolition would go relatively unremarked. The Labour Party was probably right to be ultra cautious in this respect; the power of fears about additional tax burden was amply demonstrated by the run-up to and the result of the 1992 election, and it is probably not unfair to suggest that only a party confident that it stands no chance of being elected would have the temerity to propose the outright abolition of MITR.

There was one further major difference between the opposition parties. Both had positive proposals for a revival of rented housing, which they both saw as an urgent necessity, but they seriously differed as to which agency should be largely responsible for the provision of rented housing. The Liberal Democrats preferred to go for the subsidised 'new' sector of Partnership Housing, largely consisting of 'mutual societies' as landlords, while the Labour Party preferred to return to the tried and tested ground of local authorities as landlords. To that end, the Labour Party proposed that the funding of council housing be returned to the pre-1988 deficit funding system whereby central government made up the shortfall between rental income and expenditure on housing revenue account; a similar system of deficit funding was to be reintroduced for housing associations. They also proposed to remove the obligation on councils to charge capital-value-based rents, and instead proposed that rents be based on a 'reasonable' proportion of the local level of manual wages. Moreover, the 'ring-fencing' of housing revenue accounts was to come to an end (a proposal that the Liberal Democrats positively opposed), and it would no longer be necessary for council tenants to fund local housing benefit expenditure or local rent arrears. The Labour Party was clearly taking the view that council housing was a community responsibility and that council tenants should not bear all the costs of its provision:

> The local authority's general fund (as distinct from the housing revenue account) will pay for all services, including some housing services, that serve the whole community. . . . It will be possible for contributions to be made from the general fund to the housing revenue account, as local authorities will be held to account for such contributions by the local electorate as a whole.
>
> (Labour Party 1991f: 14)

In other respects these parties' policies were much closer to each other, particularly in their views about owner occupation. Neither party wanted to hurt owner occupiers, but both wanted to ensure that those who found it expensive to enter owner occupation were helped to do so, and equally those who wished to exit from it were also assisted. Thus both proposed a 'mortgage to rent' scheme to help owner occupiers in trouble, and methods to reduce the trans-action costs of buying and selling through, for example, introducing 'log books' for property; the Liberal Democrats proposed to abolish stamp duty on house purchase. Neither proposed to abandon the 'right to buy'.

Thus the main way in which the parties were similar, and at the same time differed from the Conservative Party, was that they saw a strong place for a subsidised rented sector, and wanted what both parties now called 'social housing' to expand considerably.

Moreover, and this is particularly important as far as squaring the circle is concerned, both parties saw capital receipts from the sale of council housing as remaining part of a housing budget and available for new expenditure for building for rent. They both proposed that the restrictions on local authority spending their capital receipts be progressively lifted and that a centrally controlled credit approval system be introduced for those authorities wishing to borrow to build. The Labour Party, following a recently published Fabian Society pamphlet (Merrett and Cranston 1992), proposed to institutionalise this claim to capital receipts as available for housing investment by establishing a National Housing Bank where local authorities with high capital receipts could make deposits and then receive market rates of interest; the Bank would then lend out the money to any organisation, including private landlords, wishing to build for rent. Such a move would apparently be anathema to the Conservative Party, since it would encourage new investment in housing by local authorities, and give them back some considerable power over their own finances. At the same time, the use of these monies for capital investment would seriously decrease the amount available to repay debt, thus increasing the Public Sector Borrowing Requirement, and decrease the investment income of local authorities. Both Labour and Liberal Democrats, working within the discourses both of economic management and of need, were clearly of the opinion that the use of these monies would stimulate demand and hence growth, and this would outweigh the short-term revenue costs.

HOUSING POLITICS IN THE 1990s

It is possible to argue, therefore, that there are elements both of consensus and of dissensus among the three main political parties concerning housing. All three accept that owner occupation should remain the tenure housing the vast majority of British households, that routes into that tenure should be made easier through, for example, maintaining the 'right to buy' of council tenants and reducing some elements of transaction costs, and that mortgagors should have financial assistance either through the indiscriminate and regressive MITR, or, as the Liberal Democrats suggest, through targeted assistance to owners on low incomes. The difference between the parties lies in their attitude as to whether there has to be a limit to the expansion of owner occupation, and to that end, whether a firm basis for the further development of rented housing has to be established now. Here the Labour Party and Liberal Democrats are in agreement: both acknowledge that renting must be developed, and not just for a stigmatised or transient minority. While both Labour and Liberal Democrat manifestos referred to 'social housing', it is nevertheless clear that the Labour Party continues to prefer the traditional route to rented housing via central government deficit funding of local authorities, while the Liberal Democrats wish to see a new form of landlordism develop, subsidised both by producer and consumer subsidies.

Despite the radical changes in the housing system brought about by the Conservatives under Thatcher, it is clear that one of the great successes of Conservative housing strategy in the 1980s was to bring the discourse of ownership into absolute pre-dominance. It is possible that, even in a situation of continuous high real interest rates, owner occupation will remain relatively stable and attractive to the huge majority of households and hence that discourse may well prevail, to the Conservatives' considerable electoral advantage, into the 1990s. Much depends on how far – to use John Major's phrase – the 'cascades of wealth down the generations' act to cushion the households on the edge of viability, rather than simply act to increase demand for owner occupation and thus increase the price of entry. But there are other factors already in place which might feed a new politics of housing policy within the Conservative Party itself: the question whether there are elements within Conservative policy which will lead to intolerable tension such that it will be forced to change direction; the question as to whether the Conservatives, with a considerably smaller majority than during the 1980s, will be rather more sensitive to public opinion, and, with that, the question as to what public opinion is likely to do about housing; the question of the attitude of local governments to housing finance and whether or not they will exert effective pressure on central government to change direction.

There is a distinct possibility that there is now so much volatility in the owner-occupied sector that it will eventually force a change of direction either within that party itself, or possibly at the ballot box. One way of dealing with the intrinsic vulnerability and volatility of mass owner occupation is to develop a view that there is a limit to the expansion of the tenure; that it is not suitable, particularly in a situation of high interest rates, for a substantial minority of the population, and that some viable alternative tenure in the form of renting has to be developed. There are signs that such a view is beginning to take hold in the Conservative Party (Walden 1992) and ideas of developing a new form of private landlordism using building societies as landlords are being seriously considered (*Independent on Sunday*, 2 August 1992). However, such proposals would not be cost free; in order to maintain a rate of return on renting such that would attract building societies, who have to pay competitive interest rates to their depositors, such tenancies would entail substantial transfers, either in the form of Housing Benefit to tenants, or of subsidies to these new landlords – possibly through the tax system. A Treasury determined to maintain low public expenditure may prefer to rely on the traditional market system for private renting. But unfortunately for the Treasury, there is plenty of evidence that deregulated rents in the private sector *high* enough to provide a competitive investment opportunity, particularly at a time when the long-term capital growth potential of residential property is apparently in decline, are, at the same time, unlikely to be *low* enough to attract effective demand from owner occupiers currently in financial difficulty. There is no doubt that the Treasury will at some point have to try to resolve the problem as to how to maintain the housing system, and the economic system with it, while at the same time holding a very tight rein on subsidies in the housing system. In my view, such a juggling act is not possible; if the rented sector is to house, in sufficient numbers, those households for whom owner occupation is currently proving to be a quagmire both for themselves and for the British economy, then there will have to be significant subsidy to the rented sector, routed through consumers, or producers, or both.

There are further difficulties on the horizon to do with public opinion. During the 1992 election campaign a MORI poll commissioned by Shelter found that 91 per cent of the sample thought housing and homelessness a serious problem in contemporary Britain, placing it above health (69 per cent) and education (77 per cent) in their list of concerns (Dwelly 1992). But these were questions couched only within the needs discourse. It is therefore interesting to note that, during the very same election campaign, none of the parties thought housing need and policy a topic worthy of attention since, presumably, they thought the needs discourse extremely weak at the time. Only Michael Heseltine managed to hit the headlines by prophesying a further drop in house prices if Labour enacted its tax plans, and, if Labour were elected, a hike in interest rates which would adversely affect all mortgagors.

Heseltine was right to play on these anxieties for short-term Conservative advantage. As a result of owner occupation becoming the mass tenure, interest rates policy is now of personal interest to the mass of electors; the whole question of macro money management is now highly politicised as the extraordinary events of 16 September 1992, when Britain fell out of the ERM, demonstrate. While Britain's exit from the ERM has brought a small, but possibly only temporary reprieve from very high interest rates, a government committed to control of the money supply as the major weapon against inflation is in a very difficult position – politically, financially, and economically. The only defence in its armoury to protect owner occupiers from high interest rates is MITR. But this is a singularly ineffective way of defending the living standards of those most vulnerable to interest rate increases since this tax subsidy makes no distinction between those on first or subsequent mortgages, and those on high or low incomes. Moreover, MITR is a very expensive tax expenditure; and if it proves too difficult to do away with it, or radically alter it, for political reasons, then it will not quickly 'wither on the vine' (IBH 1991: 37). Thus the fact that MITR is so unselective renders it both expensive and ineffective at protecting those most vulnerable – a point that all Conservatives should find particularly easy to understand. Yet it is the lower-income households who actually keep the owner-occupied housing market in business; if they fail to form or maintain themselves as households, the whole market, dependent as it is on chains of buyers and sellers, is vulnerable if not to collapse, then at least to stasis. And with that, as we have already argued, comes the possible stasis of the whole of the British economy. At some point, it seems inevitable that the nettle of indiscriminate and regressive nature of MITR will have to be tackled – if not for reasons of equity, then for reasons of economic management.

But it is not only conflicts within the Treasury which are likely to bring considerable stress and strain to Conservative policies. The Departments of Trade and Industry and of Environment are also likely to be pulled into the fray. For example, the

Conservative intention remains that the housing subsidies that exist should much more predominantly aid consumers than producers; in other words, Housing Benefit should be the tenants' bulwark against hardship rather than rent regulation in the private sector, or generous exchequer grants and loans at low interest in the social sector. But, as we have already seen, there are real difficulties with the Housing Benefit system; in many cases it amounts to an expensive way of delivering housing that is free at the point of consumption to the unemployed, and a way of entrapping the low paid in poverty. The effect of this is that those urban areas with high proportions of tenants will also contain high proportions of households trapped in poverty by means-tested benefits. In other words, this policy of consumer subsidies has a spatial effect as well as a social effect. The really strong spatial effect will occur on those council estates which are least popular and which local housing departments customarily use as 'dumping grounds' for their most stigmatised tenants – those coming through the homelessness route to rehousing, those on very low per capita incomes or dependent on Income Support. The 1992 Conservative manifesto promised that the management of council estates would be put out to competitive tendering by private management companies (later confirmed in the Queen's speech). Part of these companies' remit will be to collect the rents, so they will have a strong interest in ensuring that the bulk of their tenants are on Income Support and hence have their rents paid directly by the DSS. The consequence for the government's new 'Urban Regeneration Agency', which is designed to bring employment and environmental improvement into the inner city, is that it may founder on the rock of social security targeting.

There is one further source of tension within government which may also move to the fore. One of the major planks of all Conservative social policy appears to be to remove as many powers as possible from local government. Housing has been no exception to this general rule, the most telling example being the very careful restriction of local authorities' power to spend their capital receipts accrued through the enforced sale of council housing. Local authorities are growing increasingly vociferous in their demand that control of these monies be returned to them, and that they be allowed to spend them on 'social' housing. Nevertheless, it is not absolutely clear that local housing authorities will mount a strong campaign to recover their control of these monies. Given general tightening on public expenditure, it is in the interests of all authorities to maintain some income to current accounts through the shrewd investment of their enforced savings. Thus the political pressure from this source to release these monies may in itself be weak and divided and, as public expenditure restrictions tighten into the 1990s, grow weaker.

I have argued that present Conservative housing policy is, at many levels, a recipe for political conflict. There will be tensions within and between government departments and between central and local government. If the opposition parties do their job properly they should be able to exploit these tensions – and they have alternative strategies already developed, if not costed. The dominance of the ownership discourse which has proved such an electoral advantage for the Conservatives may well have had its heyday; it is very possible that the 1990s will see a return to the discourses of needs and of economic management.

Moreover, the question of what constitutes housing 'need' may in itself become more and more politicised. It is interesting to note that when a system moves increasingly into the private sector, as the housing system has done since the 1970s and, with increasing speed, in the 1980s, then an engine of household fission is put in place. A private market has no interest in depressing household fission – indeed quite the reverse – since new household formation creates further demand which helps to construct a system dependent on first-time buyers for its ultimate maintenance. This applies both to the market for second-hand and for new housing. But once such new households start to form, whether they are elderly people, very young adults, people with special needs, single people of all ages with and without children, or married couples who wish to live separately from each other, the prevailing expectations of what constitutes a legitimate 'household' start to change. This process underlies the, as yet, unfulfilled demand that the homelessness legislation should apply to single people without children, and without special needs – a demand which the Labour Party intends, eventually, to meet. In other words, the private sector capitalist engine of developing new 'needs' spills over into the public sector, which, subject to scarce resources, in its turn seeks to depress 'need'. The way in which this contradiction is resolved feeds the politics of housing policy, and creates, for the remaining public sector of housing provision, a particular problem of squaring the circle. It seems that, during the 1990s, housing policy will be subject to very considerable stresses and strains, for both political and macro-economic reasons.

Chapter 10

2000 and beyond
A residual or a citizens' welfare state?

Vic George and Stewart Miller

In this final chapter, we concentrate on two key conclusions that emerge from the foregoing chapters and which have clear and significant implications for the future development of the welfare state.

The first conclusion is that, as the main political parties stand in the early 1990s and as they are likely to develop during this decade, the similarities between their policies are at least as important as their differences. This is not to say that their day-to-day differences are negligible; it is evident that they are not. But the central assumptions of policy are largely shared by the parties; they do not stray beyond the bounds of what we have called the affordable welfare state.

On the economic front, they are all committed to a largely privately-owned economy, constantly pursuing higher rates of economic growth, beating down inflation rather than maintaining full employment, and integrating the British economy with that of the European Community, however extensive that market becomes. They disagree on the establishment of a national minimum wage, with the Conservatives insisting that this will bring financial ruin to the country despite the evidence to the contrary from countries where such a minimum has long been adopted. They also disagree somewhat on the acceptable extent of state intervention in the industrial regeneration of the country, with Labour adopting a more interventionist policy particularly in relation to industrial training. But, in general, there is no support for a return to either the large-scale public ownership or the mass subsidy of uneconomic firms that characterised policy in the pre-1980 years.

On the fiscal side, all parties are in support of low taxation on incomes, although they disagree on just how low that level should be. There is no support for a return to the high rates of the 1970s and before. The disagreements are on whether existing low personal taxation rates should be maintained, reduced slightly further, or increased to a modest degree. The Conservative Party policy for further reductions in direct taxation rates is based on the belief that these will encourage economic growth and ultimately bring in more revenue to finance services. This has always been a disputed economic theory, and the experience of this country since the major tax rate reductions of the 1980s casts further doubt on its credibility. Reviews of both national and international research have concluded that current rates of taxation have little influence, positive or negative, on rates of economic growth. The authoritative OECD study of 1975 concluded that the various types of evidence from a range of advanced industrial societies indicate:

> that taxation does not have a large and significant effect on the total supply of work effort, and that in particular the net effect on the labour supply of male family heads is likely to be very small. Moreover, there is some evidence that taxation has little influence on the choice of occupations. The empirical work available therefore tends to support (the conclusion) that the net effect of taxation on labour supply is not large enough to be of great economic or sociological significance.
>
> (Godfrey 1975: 126)

Ten years later another OECD study concluded that to date the empirical evidence 'has produced estimates of labour supply responses to taxation which are neither strong nor robust' but added significantly that despite this, 'concern over these alleged effects remains widespread' (Saunders and Klau 1985: 166). Studies of the effects of taxation rates on the propensity to save have reached very similar conclusions: that is, that levels of direct taxation have no consistent influence on the levels of national savings. These reviews referred to the relatively high direct taxation rates of the early 1980s and before and with the reduction of these rates during the late 1980s one would have logically expected the issue to have lost its party political significance. This ought to have been the case particularly in the UK, which experienced the sharpest reductions in direct taxation in the 1980s and today has one of the lowest taxation rates in the industrialised world. Government data show that among 16 OECD countries in 1989, the UK ranked tenth in terms of all taxes as percentage of GDP; it ranked joint second in terms of the significance of indirect taxes in the total volume of taxation; it ranked eighth in terms of the significance of direct taxes on households in the total volume of taxation; and it ranked thirteenth in terms of the significance of social security contributions in the total volume of taxation (CSO 1992b: 116–17). In other words, the UK was not only among the lowest taxed OECD countries but it relied on indirect taxation more than most other countries for its revenues. Objectively, there is no case for any further reductions in direct taxation.

Nevertheless, the all-party support for relatively low rates of income tax reflects the parties' interpretation of the public mood, which in turn arises from the structural imperatives of a consumption-oriented society. People have come to believe that constantly rising rates of consumption are the key to the good life and they are loath to surrender more of their income in taxes than is absolutely necessary. They seem, however, to be relatively tolerant of indirect taxes as part of the consumption process. In any case, low rates of personal taxation are now an established public expectation, and political parties wanting to expand or improve the social services find themselves having to take this into account. Indeed, the intolerance of high personal taxation is one of the central assumptions of social politics in the 1990s. It is also likely to continue, for the public appetite for consumption is constantly fostered by powerful forces in the industrial and technological systems, creating what Marcuse referred to twenty-five years ago as 'one-dimensional consumer craving personalities' (Marcuse 1968). This process seems to occur irrespective of the nature of the political system.

In the sphere of specific policy, the foregoing chapters show that the similarities between the parties are also in evidence. In housing they have all accepted, on the one hand, what Ungerson calls 'the discourse of ownership', taking private ownership to be the most valued form of tenure, worthy of encouragement by government; and on the other, the necessity for subsidies to those on low incomes to help meet their housing costs. They do disagree on the role of the social housing sector and on the detail and extent of benefit schemes. In education, they all accept that the state has a responsibility to provide universal and free schooling –

and indeed a vested interest in doing so – though they disagree as to how this should be administered and on the role, but not the existence, of private education. They all stand for the expansion of higher education – without the restoration of adequate grant support for students. In health, the NHS receives strong all-party support but there are disagreements on the role of markets and on the level of funding that will be feasible. These agreements and differences appear also in the personal social services, and there is little evidence that any party wishes to amend the contrast between the residuality of that range of services and the comprehensiveness of public health care. In social security, the parties are all committed to the two-tier pattern of insurance and assistance, though the Conservatives give greater emphasis to the role of private provision and the Liberal Democrats would like eventually to integrate the tax and benefit systems. No party has produced policies that respond effectively to the family and labour market changes of the post-war period, because of the cost implications. All in all, our conclusion that the differences between the parties' economic and social policies are contained within the common paradigm of the affordable welfare state seems well grounded.

Our second main conclusion is that if current policies continue, the affordable welfare state will gradually decline into a residual welfare state, as much by default, through inadequate funding, as through deliberate policy. At times of economic stagnation or decline – the very time when ideas of welfare state containment tend to become current – there are major problems, particularly as the demand for public services frequently rises as a consequence of economic difficulties. High rates of unemployment have manifold effects on levels of public expenditure: on one hand, they reduce government tax revenues and on the other they bolster government expenditures through the payment of benefits, retraining, and increased demand for health and social work services. It is estimated that the cost to the Exchequer, in terms of revenues lost and benefits paid, of an unemployed person is at least £8,000 per annum.

The Conservative Party has been in power for most of the period during which these problems have been most severe and the ideas of containment most prevalent. Conservative governments, on the one hand, have tried to dampen down demand for public services; to manage them in such a way as to encourage efficiency and maintain the market incentives they believe will bring about economic growth; and to keep wage rises of state employees below those in the private sector. For the eleven-year period 1979–90, the rise in the average wages of government employees was 26.6 per cent lower than the rise in the average private sector wage (Oxley and Martin 1991: 166). Even in 1992, when the Conservative Chancellor of the Exchequer tried to use public works in a halfheartedly Keynesian fashion to deliver a boost to the economy at large and the property market in particular, he also introduced an incomes policy for the public sector to protect – and indeed enhance – the savings referred to above, with the certain effect of widening the differentials between private and public sector workers.

On the other hand, Conservative governments have raised indirect taxation, sold nationalised industries and borrowed heavily from time to time, depending on the state of the economy. As we saw in Chapter 2, they have had mixed success in all this, but seem to have convinced a substantial section of the electorate that they have been doing a good job in difficult circumstances. As we pointed out in Chapter 3, however, if economic growth remains low throughout the 1990s and unemployment remains high, as appears to be the case, the Conservative Party, if it retains power, will be faced with a very difficult choice by the year 2000: in order to square the welfare circle, it will have to opt either (a) to raise money somehow or (b) to slim down the social services even more, moving from the affordable welfare state to the residual welfare state.

Both of these options for replacing the universal welfare state of the post-war period still remain open. That earlier set of arrangements was characterised by large, relatively monolithic organisations, clearly placed within the public sector and dominated by various combinations of professionals and bureaucrats. It sported a culture of public service, with all the dedication and also all the inflexibility, and all the generation of a public sector presence in social politics, that that implied. Conservative policy continues to be aimed at the fragmentation of that sector and the destruction of its collective culture. The welfare state is being prepared for either of the turn-of-the-century options. If the first is to be taken and more revenue is to be generated, the market culture which accompanies school opt-outs, the division of budget holders from service providers in health care, and agency separation from central ministries will be relied on to maintain and enhance the search for new resources. If the second option is chosen, the political context will be that the collective forces – trade unions, professional bodies, middle-class pressure groups – which might have defended the old system have been weakened, and the transition can be presented as a natural development. Where the political and administrative circumstances were favourable, the Conservatives have been tempted some way down this road already: the virtual cessation of public house-building, and the funding decisions which have led to dentists abandoning the National Health Service, are prototype policies of this kind. These and other examples lead us to the conclusion that it is this residual welfare state option that the Conservatives are likely to adopt if economic growth does not improve substantially.

The Labour Party has been trying to develop its own method of squaring the circle. Its difficulties have in some degree become greater as its period of exile from office has stretched longer and longer and the electorate's conviction of its competence in government weakened. The Labour Party has increasingly felt itself obliged to act with caution and a very constrained kind of realism, while still trying to maintain its distinctiveness from the Conservatives. Labour have argued that the development and improvement of the public services in the short term will have to be slight and capable of being financed by modest increases in the progressiveness of direct taxation. In the long run, Labour accept the 'affordability axiom' that further improvements are dependent on improved economic performance. Its vision of the good society still seems to resemble a fully developed universalist welfare state; but how much of this can, or even should, be defended is a matter under debate. The party is conscious not only of the need for credibility now but of its past experience in government, with its many forced compromises and departures from its declared values.

If anything, the agonising of the Labour Party was further stimulated by the result of the 1992 General Election, in which the voters appeared to reject the modest increases in taxation which the party proposed, despite popular criticisms of the Conservatives' handling of the welfare services. Labour have to establish whether this apparent public unwillingness to pay higher taxes is indeed real, and so firmly embedded in British society that there is no point in persevering with any such policy; or whether, with new leadership and better presentation of policy, enough of the electorate can be won over. If it reaches the first conclusion, then it has to reformulate its method of squaring the welfare circle. It has to find ways of raising more revenue, reducing service costs, or both. Labour could find itself, in office in the late 1990s, faced with the same dilemma we have already described for the Conservatives. This could also be the case if Labour were to reach a more optimistic conclusion about the political viability of raising taxes but came to power after a prolonged period of recession presided over by the Conservatives. And even if Labour came to office prepared to raise taxation or borrowing or both, the one option it could not take up would be that of reproducing the post-war version of the welfare state. Market culture, the demands of consumerism, higher general standards of living, new patterns of need and the effects of a long period of Conservatism would preclude the inflexibility and the lack of choice and accountability associated with that model. In any case, there is little evidence in the early 1990s that Labour is ready to shake off the caution and orthodoxy which characterised the period of Neil Kinnock's leadership and which seem to be inherent traits of John Smith and his advisers.

The Liberal Democrats, meanwhile, are faced with the problem of maintaining their distinctiveness and their influence in national politics. The 1992 election demonstrated how improbable are the circumstances in which the Liberal Democrats can hope to influence policy in the present system, and it may be that their role will be essentially that of a pressure group for constitutional change rather than an active participant in the politics of squaring the welfare circle.

Advanced industrial societies provide the kind of welfare states that, politically, they *will*. This is no less true in the face of the economic and other difficulties we have discussed, for the wealth of such countries is still immense. What distinguishes welfare state laggards from others is not so much lack of resources as lack of political will to go further – or, more assertively, a distinct aversion to the growth and development of state welfare. The USA is one of the most affluent among OECD countries but also one of the lowest welfare state spenders; Portugal, with a considerably lower income per capita, spends a greater proportion of its GDP on public services. If Britain in the 1990s and 2000s used its resources differently – if it deployed them on a different set of political assumptions – it could provide a welfare system as comprehensive as Beveridge's vision, although its forms would no doubt be quite different. What would be required would be not only a shift in the assumptions of governments but also a shift in the public attitudes; the two relate to each other through feedback loops. We refer to such an alternative to residualism as a citizens' welfare state, not only because it would be characterised by an institutional concern to preserve the welfare entitlements of citizenship, but because its viability is so highly dependent on the will of the people.

Much has been said about the influence of public opinion on government policies and far less on the influence that governments can exert on shaping public opinion. Governments that want to maintain even the affordable welfare state will need to concentrate some of their efforts in educating the public that social services are worth paying for, not only for self-interest reasons but on grounds of efficiency and community. Countries which neglect their social services neglect at the same time their future economic prosperity and their social cohesion and stability. Social and economic policy are interdependent and neither is superior to the other in terms of the welfare of the public. This view of social and economic policy is not confined to the left but cuts across party political boundaries in this country. Pym, representing the traditional Tory view, expressed it very well when he said that 'social policy should never be subservient to economic policy' but always bearing in mind that national wealth has to be created to provide the finance for social policy expenditure (Pym 1985: 129).

Despite this bipartisan view on the merits of social policy, most 'establishment' commentators on how to square the welfare circle in the future put forward proposals which involve further reductions in expenditure and services rather than increases in service revenues and provisions. The new right view that public expenditure is a drain on economic resources has become the conventional wisdom and permeates most thinking on the future of welfare. In their review of public expenditure in the 1980s in OECD countries, Oxley and Martin conclude that the way to square the welfare circle in the 1990s is not through increased revenues, for the prospects are bleak, but through continuing the policies of trimming, charging and restructuring that were initiated in the 1980s. The reasons why the prospects for increased revenues are bleak are not only the poor prospects for economic growth but also the view that increased taxation is undesirable on economic as well as political grounds. They therefore propose more of the same – specifically, three broad policies:

> i) increasing efficiency in the delivery of government goods and services and in programme efficacy; ii) reviewing spending priorities and programme objectives; and iii) devolving some public responsibilities to the private sector.
>
> (Oxley and Martin 1991: 178)

No one can in principle argue against increased efficiency but one can both question the extent to which further improvements in true efficiency are possible: and one can also raise the often neglected issue that increased efficiency in the public services has been achieved partly at the expense of the living standards of those who work in these services. Reviewing spending priorities is an enigmatic way of dealing with the problem, for every population group can argue that the axe should fall on some service that benefits some other group rather than itself. There are, however, instances when a rational case can be put forward for reducing expenditure in a particular area because of a radically changed situation. Defence expenditure is one such instance in view of the political changes in Eastern Europe. Among OECD countries, the UK ranks second to the USA in terms of defence expenditure as a percentage of GDP and it is now generally accepted that expenditure reductions in this area are necessary. The peace dividend, however, may not be as great as it is often thought, not only because of political reasons but also because, in a period of recession, reductions in army personnel may only increase the numbers of unemployment benefit recipients. As for the third policy proposal of devolving yet more areas of public policy to the private sector, experience has shown that those most in need tend to lose out. The net result of this set of proposals is a gradual shift towards the residual welfare state.

Proposals for squaring the welfare circle reflect political as well as economic considerations. Those who view the prospects of a residual welfare state with alarm and who may go as far as supporting a citizens' welfare state have to accept that, in the likely event of low rates of economic growth in the future, their proposals mean higher rates of indirect or direct taxation. Some aspects of the citizens' welfare state involve no higher expenditure but others do. The participatory, empowering aspects of a citizens' welfare state are in tune with contemporary public attitudes, have no cost implications and receive support from all political parties. However, this only deals with the issue of procedural rights in welfare and not with the question of substantive rights which is at the heart of the notion of a citizens' welfare state. The notion of substantive rights implies that people have quasi-legalistic entitlements in some areas of welfare and hard legal entitlements in others but in all areas they can expect a level of benefits and services that goes beyond the current levels of provision. It may be possible to raise some of the necessary extra funds through some reallocation of spending priorities but, as mentioned above, this will be neither easy nor sufficient. Governments may borrow to finance a citizens' welfare state but again this cannot be done indefinitely. The issue of higher taxation comes back to haunt the proponents of a citizens' welfare state for, in view of the state of the economy, there is no other way of squaring their welfare circle in the immediate future.

In 1992 the forced withdrawal from the European exchange rate mechanism, the subsequent devaluation of sterling, the crisis in the coal industry and public reaction to it and the realisation that Conservative governments in such countries as Germany and Japan were using Keynesian strategies to combat recession undermined the monetarist view of the damaging effects of public expenditure on economic growth and led to a limited adoption of Keynesianism in this country too. The argument that, on the contrary, public expenditure is an essential ingredient of the economic mix of a modern society was reasserted in new forms. As the limitations of unbounded Keynesianism were exposed in the late 1970s, so were those of rampant monetarism in the early 1990s. There is a better understanding now that neither orthodoxy, in a pure form, can sustain the health of a modern economy.

This new pragmatic economic thinking provides a better climate for halting and perhaps reversing the drift of the affordable welfare state into residualism. For a long time the Conservative Party has been playing all the tunes, and the opposition, if not dancing to them, is at least showing no fundamental dissent. Labour and the Liberal Democrats – and indeed the 'one nation' wing of Toryism – now have an opportunity to influence if not to determine the agenda around the nature of the welfare state. It is open to the Labour and Liberal Democratic Parties to make the case for a change of direction away

from residualism and towards comprehensiveness, on the twin
arguments of a positive economic role for public expenditure and
public support for improved services. The argument could not be
for a return to the bureaucratic model of post-war welfare, but for
a forward move towards an empowering, efficient and
comprehensive citizens' welfare state. Nor could they avoid the
difficult task of convincing the electorate that such a welfare state
needs to be adequately financed. It might be the case that
ear-marked taxes, as we have at present in social security, would
have a new and wider role in bringing home to the public the
connection between the provision of good quality public services
and their funding. There is a strong democratic case for giving the
public the choice between a residual welfare state with low taxes
and a citizens' welfare state at a higher tax cost before the former
wins out by default on the assumption that it is the only way of
squaring the welfare circle.

Bibliography

Abel-Smith, B. and Townsend, P. (1965) *The Poor and the Poorest*. London: Bell.

Adler, M. and Sainsbury, R. (1991) 'Administrative justice, quality of service and the operational strategy' in Adler, M. and Williams, R. (eds) *The Social Implications of the Operational Strategy*. New Working Papers, Social Policy Series No.4, University of Edinburgh.

Alcock, P. (1991) 'Towards welfare rights' in Becker, S. (ed.) *Windows of Opportunity: Public Policy and the Poor* per cent0. London: Child Poverty Action Group.

Anderton, B., Britton, A. and Soteri, S. (1991) 'The home economy.' *National Institute Economic Review*, 136, May, 10–26.

Ashdown, P. (1990/1) 'Breaking the poverty trap: a basic income.' *Basic Income Research Group Bulletin* 12.

Atkinson, A. and Micklewright, J. (1988) *Turning the Screw: Benefits for the Unemployed 1979–1988*, Discussion Paper No. TIDI/121. London: Suntory-Toyota International Centre for Economics and Related Disciplines.

Audit Commission (1992) *Developing Local Authority Housing Strategies*. London: HMSO.

Bacon, R. and Eltis, W.A. (1976) *Britain's Economic Problem: Too Few Producers*. London: Macmillan.

Baldwin-Edwards, M. and Gough, I. (1991) 'EC social policy and the UK' in Manning, N. (ed.) *Social Policy Review 1990–91*. Harlow: Longman.

Ball, M., Gray, F. and McDowell, L. (1989) *The Transformation of Britain*. London: Fontana.

Barbour, R.S. (1989) 'Health and illness.' *Developments in Sociology* 7: 105–29.

Barnett, R.R., Levaggi, R. and Smith, P. (1990) 'The impact of party politics on patterns of service provision in English local authorities.' *Policy and Politics* 18 (3): 217–29.

Barr, N. and Coulter, F. (1990) 'Social security: solution or problem?' in Hills, J. (ed.) *The State of Welfare: The Welfare State in Britain since 1974*. Oxford: Clarendon Press.

Bazen, S. and Thirlwall, T. (1989) *Deindustrialisation*. London: Heinemann.

Bellaby, P. (1977) *The Sociology of Comprehensive Schooling*. London: Methuen.

Bennett, F. (1991) 'A window of opportunity' in Becker, S. (ed.) *Windows of Opportunity: Public Policy and the Poor*. London: Child Poverty Action Group.

Bennington, J. (1991) *The Integration of the EMU*. Report. York: Joseph Rowntree Foundation.

Blackaby, F. (ed.) (1979) *Deindustrialisation*. London: Heinemann.

Blanchflower, D.G. and Oswald, A.J. (1990) 'Self-employment and the enterprise culture' in Jowell *et al*. (eds) *British Social Attitudes: The Seventh Report*. Aldershot: Gower.

Bleaney, M. (1985) *The Rise and Fall of Keynesian Economics*. London: Macmillan.

Blunkett, D. (1991) *Retirement or Rejection: The Challenge and Opportunity of Ageing*. London: Labour Party.

Board of Inland Revenue (1990) *Inland Revenue Statistics, 1990*. London: HMSO.

Booth, C. (1902) *The Life and Labour of the London Poor: Volume 1: Poverty*. London: Macmillan.

Bottomley, V. (1992) 'Building on a solid state.' *Community Care*, 2 April: 19–20.

Brindle, D. (1992) 'Analysis: the effects of inflation, medical advances and an ageing population offer little comfort to Labour.' *Guardian*, 25 March.

Brittan, S. (1975) 'The economic contradictions of democracy.' *British Journal of Political Science* 5(1).

—— (1977) 'Can democracy manage an economy?' in Skidelsky, R. (ed.) *The End of the Keynesian Era*. London: Macmillan.

Brown, J. (1990) 'The focus on single mothers' in Murray, C. *et al*. *The Emerging British Underclass*. London: Institute of Economic Affairs.

Bucknall, B. (ed.) (1991) *Housing Finance*, 2nd edition. London: CIPFA.

Cairncross, A. (1992) *The British Economy Since 1945: Economic Policy and Performance, 1945–1990*. Oxford: Blackwell.

Central Statistical Office (CSO) (1984) *Social Trends No. 14*. London: HMSO.

—— (1987) *Social Trends No. 17*. London: HMSO.

—— (1991) *Social Trends No. 21*. London: HMSO.

—— (1992a) *Social Trends No. 22*. London: HMSO.

—— (1992b) 'International comparison of taxes and social security contributions in 20 OECD countries, 1979–1989.' *Economic Trends* 459.

Clarke, K. (1992) 'Sixth form schooling.' *Press Release*, February.

Cochrane, A.L. (1972) *Effectiveness and Efficiency: Random Reflections on Health Services*. London: Nuffield Provincial Hospitals Trust.

Coleman, D. and Salt, J. (1992) *The British Population: Patterns, Trends and Processes*. Oxford: Oxford University Press.

Conservative Party (1979) *The Conservative Manifesto 1979*. London: Conservative Central Office.

—— (1983) *The Conservative Manifesto 1983*. London: Conservative Central Office.

—— (1987) *Our First Eight Years: The Achievements of the Conservative Government since May 1979*. London: Conservative Central Office.

—— (1989) *Attacks Answered. A Politics Today Special*. London: Conservative Research Department.

—— (1990) *Politics Today 3: Employment and Industrial Relations*. Foreword by Michael Howard. London: Conservative Research Department.

—— (1991) *Labour's Public Expenditure Plans*. London: Conservative Party.

—— (1992) *The Best Future for Britain: The Conservative Manifesto 1992*. London: Conservative Central Office.

—— (n.d.) *Conservative Policy Points*. London: Conservative Central Office.

Cook, D. (1989) *Rich Law, Poor Law*. Milton Keynes: Open University Press.

Cook, R. (1990) *A Fresh Start for Health*. London: Labour Party.

—— (1991a) *The Better Way to a Healthy Britain*. London: Labour Party.

—— (1991b) Speech to the Labour Conference, Brighton, quoted in Harman, H. (1992) *NHS: The Three-fold Tory Threat. Underfunding, Commercialisation, Privatisation*. London: Labour Party: 8.

Cooke, A. (1989) *Margaret Thatcher*. London: Aurum Press.

Coutts, K. and Godley, W. (1989) 'The British economy under Mrs Thatcher.' *Political Quarterly* 10: 137–51.

Cox, C. and Dyson, A. (1971) *The Black Papers in Education*. London: Davis Poynter.

Crafts, N.F.R. and Woodward, N. (eds) (1991) *The British Economy Since 1945*. Oxford: Clarendon Press.

Craig, J. (1983) 'The growth of the elderly population.' *Population Trends*, 32, OPCS. London: HMSO: 28–33.

Crosland, A. (1974) *Socialism Now*. London: Cape.

Crosland, S. (1982) *Tony Crosland*. London: Cape.

Culyer, A.J. (1990) 'Cost containment in Europe' in *Health Care Systems in Transition: The Search for Efficiency*. OECD Social Policy Studies 7. Paris: OECD: 29–40.

Daly, M. (1991) 'The 1980s: a decade of growth in enterprise. Self-employment data from the Labour Force Survey.' *Employment Gazette* 99 (3): 109–34.

Davies, G. (1985) *Governments Can Affect Employment: A Critique of Monetarism, Old and New*. London: Employment Institute.

Davis, C.M. (1990) 'National health services, resources constraints and shortages' in Manning, N. and Ungerson, C. (eds) *Social Policy Review 1989–90*. London: Longman: 141–68.

Day, P. and Klein, R. (1991) 'Britain's health care experiment.' *Health Affairs* 10(3): 39–59.

Deacon, A. (1991) 'The retreat from state welfare' in Becker, S. (ed.) *Windows of Opportunity: Public Policy and the Poor*. London: Child Poverty Action Group.

Dean, H. (1988/9) 'Disciplinary partitioning and the privatisation of social security.' *Critical Social Policy* 24 (8), No.3.

—— (1991) *Social Security and Social Control*. London: Routledge.

Dean, H. and Taylor-Gooby, P. (1992) *Dependency Culture: The Explosion of a Myth*. Hemel Hempstead: Harvester Wheatsheaf.

Department for Education (DfE) (1992) *Choice and Diversity: A New Framework for Schools*, Cm 2021. London: HMSO.

Department of Education and Science (DES) (1977) *Education in Schools*, Cmnd 6069. London: HMSO.
—— (1989) *Education Statistics for the UK*. London: HMSO.
—— (1992a) *The Government's Expenditure Plans, 1992–93 to 1994–95: Departmental Report*, Cm 1911. London: HMSO.
—— (1992b) *Curriculum Organisation and Classroom Practice in Primary Schools*. London: HMSO.
Department of Employment (DE) (1990) *Economic Trends*, May. London: HMSO.
—— (1991) 'Labour force trends: the next decade.' *Employment Gazette* 99(5), May: 269–80.
Department of Environment (DoE) (1977) *Housing Policy: A Consultative Document*, Cm 6851. London: HMSO.
—— (1987a) *Housing: The Government's Proposals*. London: HMSO.
—— (1987b) *The New Grant System*. London: HMSO.
—— (1988) *1985-Based Estimates of Numbers of Households in England, the Regions, Counties, Metropolitan Districts and London Boroughs 1985–2001*. London: HMSO.
—— (1992) *Housing and Construction Statistics, 1981–1991*. London: HMSO.
Department of Health (DoH) (1973, 1982, 1990) *Health and Personal Social Services Statistics*. London: HMSO.
—— (1989) *Working for Patients*, Cm 555. London: HMSO.
—— (1990) *Key Indicators of Local Authority Social Services 1988/9*. London: HMSO.
—— (1991a) *Patterns and Outcomes in Child Placement*. London: HMSO.
—— (1991b) *The Health of the Nation: a Consultative Document for Health*, Cm 1523. London: HMSO.
—— (1992) *The Patient's Charter*. London: HMSO.
Department of Health and Office of Population Censuses and Surveys (DoH and OPCS) (1992) *The Government's Expenditure Plans 1992–93: Departmental Report*, Cm 1913. London: HMSO.
Department of Health and Social Security (DHSS) (1976) *Priorities for Health and Social Services*. London: HMSO.
—— (1981) *Public Expenditure on the Social Services: Reply by the Government to the Third Report of the Select Committee on Social Services, Session 1980–81*, Cm 8464. London: HMSO.
—— (1982) *Social Security Operational Strategy: A Framework for the Future*. London: HMSO.
—— (1985) *The Reform of Social Security Vol.1*, Cm 9517. London: HMSO.
Department of Social Security (DSS) (1990a) *Households Below Average Income*. London: DSS.
—— (1990b) *Social Security Statistics 1989*. London: HMSO.
—— (1991a) *Social Security Statistics 1990*. London: HMSO.
—— (1991b) *The Government's Expenditure Plans 1991–92 to 1993–94: Departmental Report*, Cm 1514. London: HMSO.
—— (1992) *The Government's Expenditure Plans 1992–93 to 1994–95*, Cm 1914. London: HMSO.
Departments of Health, Social Security, Wales and Scotland (1989)

Caring for People: Community Care in the Next Decade and Beyond, Cm 849. London: HMSO.

Derbyshire, M.E. (1987) 'Statistical rationale for grant-related expenditure assessment (GREA) concerning personal social services.' *Journal of the Royal Statistical Society*, 150A.

Digby, A. (1989) *British Welfare Policy: Workhouse to Workforce*. London: Faber.

Ditch, J. (1991) 'The making of European social policy: developments leading to the European Social Charter' in Manning, N. (ed.) *Social Policy Review 1990–91*. Harlow: Longman.

Donnison, D. (1970) Extract from *Second Report of the Public Schools Commission* in Maclure, S. (ed.) *Educational Documents*. London: Methuen.

—— (1991a) *The New Poverty and its Implications*. Paper presented to Anglo-German Social Policy Conference, Nottingham University.

—— (1991b) *A Radical Agenda: After the New Right and the Old Left*. London: Rivers Oram Press.

Dwelly, T. (1992) 'A poll that counts.' *Roof*, May/June.

Edgell, S. and Duke, V. (1991) *A Measure of Thatcherism: A Sociology of Britain*. London: HarperCollins.

Enthoven, A.C. (1985) *Reflections on the Management of the National Health Service: An American looks at incentives to efficiency in health services management in the UK*. Occasional Papers 5. London: Nuffield Provincial Hospitals Trust.

—— (1990) 'What can Europeans learn from Americans?' in *Health Care Systems in Transition: The Search for Efficiency*. OECD Social Policy Studies No.7. Paris: OECD: 57–71.

—— (1991) 'Internal Market Reform of the British NHS.' *Health Affairs* 10(3): 60–70.

Ermisch, J. (1990) *Fewer Babies, Longer Lives: Policy Implications of Current Demographic Trends*. York: Joseph Rowntree Foundation.

Esping-Anderson, G. (1990) *The Three Worlds of Welfare Capitalism*. Cambridge: Polity Press.

Evandrou, M. (1990) *Equity in Health and Social Care*. London: Suntory-Toyota International Centre for Economics and Related Disciplines, London School of Economics.

Evandrou, M., Falkingham, J. and Glennerster, H. (1990) 'The personal social services: everyone's poor relation but nobody's baby' in Hills, J. (ed.) *The State of Welfare: The Welfare State in Britain Since 1974*. Oxford: Clarendon Press.

Fabian Group (1978) *Deserting the Middle Ground: Tory Social Policies*. London: Fabian Society.

Falkingham, J. (1989) 'Dependency and ageing in Britain.' *Journal of Social Policy* 18(2), April: 211–33.

Family Policy Studies Centre (FPSC) (1986) *Fact Sheet 3: One Parent Families*. London: FPSC.

Fielding, N. (1990) 'The Thatcher Audit.' *New Statesman and Society*, 21 and 28 December: 20–4.

Finch, J. (1989) *Family Obligations and Social Change*. Oxford: Polity Press.

—— (1992) 'State responsibility and family responsibility for financial support in the 1990s' in ESRC *Income Security in Britain: A Research and Policy Agenda For the Next Ten Years*. London: ESRC.

Finch, J. and Mason, J. (1990) 'Filial obligations and kin support for elderly people.' *Ageing and Society* 10: 151–76.

Flynn, R. (1988) 'Political acquiescence, privatisation and residualisation in British housing policy.' *Journal of Social Policy* 17: 289–312.

Forrester, K. and Ward, K. (eds) (1991) *Unemployment, Education and Training: Case Studies from North America and Europe*. Sacramento, CA: Caddo Gap Press.

Forster, W. (1870) 'Speech introducing Elementary Education Bill, House of Commons' in Maclure, S. (ed.1986) *Educational Documents*. London: Methuen.

Fowler, N. (1984) Speech by the then Secretary for Social Services to the Joint Social Services Annual Conference, 27 September.

Friedman, M. (1962) *Capitalism and Freedom*. Chicago: Chicago University Press.

Garside, W. (1980) *The Measurement of Unemployment: Methods and Sources 1850–1979*. Oxford: Blackwell.

George, M. (1992) 'Cash for care.' *Community Care* 20: February, 9.

George, V. (1973) *Social Security and Society*. London: Routledge & Kegan Paul.

George, V. and Howards, I. (1991) *Poverty Amidst Affluence*. Cheltenham: Edward Elgar.

George, V. and Wilding, P. (1984) *The Impact of Social Policy*. London: Routledge & Kegan Paul.

Glendenning, F. and Pearson, M. (1988) *Black and Ethnic Minority Elders in Britain: Health Needs and Access to Services*. Centre for Social Gerontology, University of Keele.

Glendinning, C. and Millar, J. (1987) *Women and Poverty in Britain*. Brighton: Wheatsheaf.

Glennerster, H. and Low, W. (1990) 'Education: does it all add up?' in Hills, J. (ed.) *The State of Welfare*. Oxford: Clarendon Press.

Glynn, S. (1991) *No Alternative? Unemployment in Britain*. London: Faber.

Glynn, S. and Gospel, H. F. (1993) 'Britain's low skill equilibrium: a problem of demand.' *Industrial Relations Journal* 24(2): 113–270.

Godfrey, L. (1975) *Theoretical and Empirical Aspects of Taxation in Labour Supply*. Paris: OECD.

Gospel, H.F. (1992) *Markets, Firms, and the Management of Labour in Modern Britain*. Cambridge: Cambridge University Press.

Greenleaf, W.H. (1983) *The British Political Tradition, Vol. 2, The Ideological Inheritance*. London: Methuen.

Greve, J. (1990) *Homelessness in Britain*. London: Joseph Rowntree Trust.

Griffiths, Sir Roy (1988) *Community Care: Agenda for Action*. A report to the Secretary of State for Social Services. London: HMSO.

Guillebaud Committee (1956) *Report of the Committee of Enquiry into the Cost of the National Health Service*, Cm 9663. London: HMSO.

Heath, A.F. and McDonald, S.-K. (1987) 'Social change and the future of the left.' *Political Quarterly* 58: 364–77.

HM Senior Chief Inspector of Schools (1991) *Standards in Education, 1988–89*. London: DES.

HM Treasury (1979) *The Government's Expenditure Plans 1980–81*, Cm 7746. London: HMSO.

—— (1980) *The Government's Expenditure Plans 1980–81 to 1983–84*, Cm 7841. London: HMSO.

—— (1984) *The Next Ten Years*, Cm 9189. London: HMSO.

—— (1989) *The Government's Expenditure Plans 1989–90 to 1992–93*, Cm 621. London: HMSO.

—— (1992) *Public Expenditure Analyses to 1993/4*, Cm 1520. London: HMSO.

Habermas, J. (1975) *Legitimation Crisis*. London: Heinemann.

Hall, P. (1976) *Reforming the Welfare: The Politics of Change in the Personal Social Services*. London: Heinemann.

Harding, T. (1992) *Great Expectations . . . and Spending on Social Services*. Policy Forum Paper No. 1. London: National Institute for Social Work.

Harman, H. (1992) *NHS: The Three-fold Tory Threat. Underfunding, Commercialisation, Privatisation*. London: Labour Party.

Harris, R. (ed.) (1965) *Freedom or Free-For-All*. London: Institute of Economic Affairs.

Harris, R. and Seldon, A. (1979) *Over-Ruled on Welfare*. London: Institute of Economic Affairs.

Harrison, S., Hunter, D.J. and Pollitt, C. (1990) *The Dynamics of British Health Policy*. London: Unwin Hyman.

Hart, J. Tudor (1971) 'The "Inverse Care Law".' *The Lancet*, 27 February: 405–12.

Haskey, J. (1988) 'Recent trends in marriage and divorce and cohort analyses of the proportions of marriages ending in divorce.' *Population Trends No. 54*. London: HMSO.

Hayek, F.A. (1944) *The Road to Serfdom*. London: Routledge & Kegan Paul.

—— (1960) *The Constitution of Liberty*. London: Routledge & Kegan Paul.

—— (1978) *New Studies in Philosophy and Economics and the History of Ideas*. London: Routledge & Kegan Paul.

Haywood, A. (1992) 'A new political consensus?' *Talking Politics* 4(2), Winter.

Heath, D., Jowell, R., Curtice, J., Evans, G., Field, J. and Witherspoon, S. (1991) *Understanding Political Change: The British Voter 1964–1987*. London: Pergamon.

Hills, J. (1988) *Changing Tax*. London: Child Poverty Action Group.

Hills, J. and Mullings, B. (1990) 'Housing: a decent home for all at a price within their means' in Hills, J. (ed.) *The State of Welfare: The Welfare State in Britain since 1974*, Oxford: Clarendon Press.

House of Commons (1987) *Public Expenditure on the Social Services*, HC413. London: HMSO.

—— (1991) *Public Expenditure on Health Matters*, HC408. London: HMSO.

Hunter, D. and Wistow, G. (1991) *A Statistical Audit of Community Care*. Leeds: Nuffield Institute for Health Service Studies, Leeds University.

Hutton, W. (1992) 'Key is the dramatic plunge of public finances into the red.' *Guardian*, 11 March.

Inquiry into British Housing (IBH) (1991) *Inquiry into British Housing, Second Report*, chaired by HRH The Duke of Edinburgh. York: Joseph Rowntree Foundation.

Jenkin, P. (1980) Speech by the then Secretary of State for Health to the Conference of the Association of Directors of Social Services, 19 September.

Johnson, C. (1988) *Measuring the Economy*. London: Penguin.

—— (1991) *The Economy Under Mrs Thatcher 1979–1990*. London: Penguin.

Jones, K., Brown, J. and Bradshaw, J. (1978) *Issues in Social Policy*. London: Routledge & Kegan Paul.

Jones, R. (1987) *Wages and Employment Policy 1936–1985*. London: Allen & Unwin.

Jordan, B. (1985) *The State: Authority and Autonomy*. Oxford: Blackwell.

—— (1987) *Rethinking Welfare*. Oxford: Blackwell.

Jowell, R., Witherspoon, S. and Brook, L. (eds) (1990) *British Social Attitudes: The Seventh Report*. Social and Community Planning Research. Aldershot: Gower.

Katz, M. (1971) *Class, Bureaucracy and Schools*. New York: Praeger.

Kiernan, K. and Wicks, M. (1990) *Family Change and Future Policy*. York: Joseph Rowntree Trust.

King, A. (1975) 'Overload: problems of governing in the 1970s.' *Political Studies* XXIII, 2,3.

—— (1976) *Why is Britain Becoming Harder to Govern?* London: BBC.

Klass, A. (1975) *There's Gold in Them Thar Pills*. London: Penguin.

Kraan, R.J., Baldock, J., Davies, B., Evers, A., Johansson, L., Knapen, M., Thorslund, H. and Tunissen, C. (1991) *Care for the Elderly: Significant Innovations in Three European Countries*. Frankfurt am Main/Boulder, Colorado: Campus Verlag/Westview Press.

Labour Party (1987) *Labour Will Win*. London: Labour Party.

—— (1988) *Social Justice and Economic Efficiency. First Report of Labour's Policy Review for the 1990s*. London: Labour Party.

—— (1989) *Meet the Challenge, Make the Change: Final Report of Labour's Policy Review for the 1990s*. London: Labour Party.

—— (1990) *Looking to the Future*. London: Labour Party.

—— (1991a) *A Fresh Start for Health*. London: Labour Party.

—— (1991b) *Opportunity Britain: Labour's Better Way for the 1990s*. London: Labour Party.

—— (1991c) *Today's Education and Training: Tomorrow's Skills*. London: Labour Party.

—— (1991d) *Aiming High*. London: Labour Party.

—— (1991e) *Opportunity Britain*. London: Labour Party.

—— (1991f) *A Welcome Home: Labour's New Strategy for Housing*. London: Labour Party.

—— (1992a) *Your Good Health: A White Paper for a Labour Government*. London: Labour Party.

—— (1992b) *It's Time to Get Britain Working Again* (election manifesto). London: Labour Party.

—— (1992c) *Modernising Britain's Schools*, London: Labour Party.

Laing, W. (1991) *Empowering the Elderly: Direct Consumer Funding of Care Services*. London: Institute of Economic Affairs.

Lawson, N. (1980) *The New Conservatism*. London: Centre for Policy Studies.

Lawton, D. (1980) *The Politics of the School Curriculum*. London: Routledge & Kegan Paul.

Layard, R. (1986) *How to Beat Unemployment*. London: Employment Institute.

Le Grand, J. (1982) *The Strategy of Equality*. London: Allen & Unwin.

Lees, D. (1961) 'Health through choice' in Harris, R. (ed.) *Freedom or Free-For-All*. London: Institute of Economic Affairs.

Leontieff, W. and Duchin, F. (1985) *The Impact of Automation on Employment, 1963–2000*. Oxford: Oxford University Press.

Levitt, R. and Wall, A. (1984) *The Reorganized National Health Service*. London: Croom Helm.

Liberal Democrats (1990) *Putting Pupils First*, English Green Paper No. 3. London: Liberal Democrats.

—— (1991a) *Economics for the Future. The Liberal Democrats' Framework for Economic Policy*, Federal White Paper No. 4. London: Liberal Democrats.

—— (1991b) *Just the Job: An Immediate Programme to Reduce Unemployment*. London: Liberal Democrats.

—— (1991c) *The Price of Unemployment*. London: Liberal Democrats.

—— (1991d) *Training for Prosperity: Liberal Democratic Policies on Skills Shortages*. Policy Briefing 3. London: Liberal Democrats.

—— (1991e) Agenda for Caring. English Green Paper No. 4. London: Liberal Democrats.

—— (1992) *Changing Britain for Good: the Liberal Democrat Manifesto 1992*. Dorchester: Liberal Democrat Publications.

—— (n.d.) *Shaping Tomorrow – Starting Today*. London: Liberal Democrats.

Lister, R. (1990) *The Exclusive Society: Citizenship and the Poor*. London: Child Poverty Action Group.

Low Pay Unit (LPU) (1990a) *The New Review of the Low Pay Unit*, No.5.

—— (1990b) *The New Review of the Low Pay Unit*, No.6.

—— (1991) *The New Review of the Low Pay Unit*, No.11.

—— (1992) *The New Review of the Low Pay Unit*, No.14.

Lynes, T. (1975) 'Unemployment assistance tribunals in the 1930s' in Adler, M. and Bradley, A. (eds) *Justice, Discretion and Poverty*. Abingdon: Professional Books.

Major, J. (1991) Speech to Conservative Party Conference, 11 October 1991, published in *The Power to Choose: The Right to Own*. London: Conservative Political Centre.

Malpass, P. (1990) *Reshaping Housing Policy: Subsidies, Rents, and Residualisation*. London: Routledge.

Manning, N. (ed.) (1985) *Social Problems and Welfare Ideology*. London: Gower.

Manning, N. and Page, R. (eds) (1992) *Social Policy Review 4*. Canterbury: The Social Policy Association.

Manning, N. and Ungerson, C. (1990) *Social Policy Review 1989–90*. London: Longman.

Marcuse, H. (1968) *One-Dimensional Man*. London: Sphere Books.

Matthews, R.C.O. (1968) 'Why has Britain had full employment since the war?' *Economic Journal* 78: 555–69.

Maynard, G. (1989) 'Britain's economic revival and the balance of payments.' *Political Quarterly* 60: 152–63.

Mental Health Foundation (1990) *Mental Illness: The Fundamental Facts*. London: Mental Health Foundation.

Merrett, S. and Cranston, R. (1992) *A National Housing Bank*, Fabian Pamphlet 552. London: Fabian Society.

Meyer, J.A. (1990) 'Respondent' in *Health Care Systems in Transition: The Search for Efficiency*. OECD Social Policy Studies No.7. Paris: OECD: 115–18.

Miliband, R. (1969) *The State in Capitalist Society*. London: Weidenfeld & Nicolson.

Mishra, R. (1985) *The Welfare State in Crisis*. Brighton: Wheatsheaf.

—— (1990) *The Welfare State in Capitalist Society: Policies of Retrenchment and Maintenance in Europe, North America and Australia*. London: Harvester Wheatsheaf.

Morgan, M., Calnan, M. and Manning, N. (1985) *Sociological Approaches to Health and Medicine*. London: Croom Helm.

National Audit Office (NAO) (1991) *The Elderly: Information Requirements for Supporting the Elderly and Implications of Personal Pensions for the National Insurance Fund*. London: HMSO.

National Institute of Economic and Social Research (NIESR) (1992) *Quarterly Bulletin* (May).

Newton, T. (1991) Interview in *Poverty*, No.78.

Niner, P. and Maclennan, D. (1990) *Inquiry into British Housing: Information Notes 1990*. York: Joseph Rowntree Foundation.

Norman, A. (1986) *Triple Jeopardy: Growing Old in a Second Homeland*. London: Centre for Policy on Ageing.

Northcott, J. (1991) *Britain in 2010*. London: Policy Studies Institute.

Norwood, C. (1943) *Report of the Committee of the Secondary Schools Examination Council on Curriculum and Examinations* in Maclure, S. (ed. 1986) *Educational Documents*. London: Methuen.

O'Connor, J. (1973) *The Fiscal Crisis of the State*. London: St Martin's Press.

O'Higgins, M. (1984) 'Privatisation and Social Security.' *Political Quarterly* 55 (2).

—— (1985) 'Welfare, redistribution and inequality – disillusion, illusion and reality' in Bean, P., Feins, J. and Whynes, D. (eds) *Defence of Welfare*. London: Tavistock.

O'Sullivan, J. (1992) 'Labour "should back some Tory NHS changes".' *Independent*, 25 March.

Office of Population Censuses and Surveys (OPCS) (1989a) *The General Household Survey 1986*. London: HMSO.

—— (1989b) *The Prevalence of Disability among Children*. Bone, M. and Meltzer, H., OPCS surveys of disability in Great Britain, Report No. 3, Social Survey Division. London: HMSO.

—— (1989c) *Population Projections: Mid-1987 Based*. Monitor PP2. London: HMSO.

—— (1991) *Population Trends 66*, Winter. London: HMSO.

Oppenheim, C. (1990) *Poverty: The Facts*. London: Child Poverty Action Group.

Organisation for Economic Cooperation and Development (OECD) (1975) *Education and Working Life*. Paris: OECD.

—— (1988) *Ageing Populations*. Paris: OECD.

—— (1989) *OECD Economic Surveys – UK*. Paris: OECD.

—— (1990a) *Economic Outlook* No. 47, June. Paris: OECD.

—— (1990b) *Health Care Systems in Transition: The Search for Efficiency*. Paris: OECD.

—— (1991) 'Country report: the UK.' *Economic Outlook* No. 49, July. Paris: OECD.

—— (1992) *Economic Outlook* No. 51, June. Paris: OECD.

Oxley, H. and Martin, J.P. (1991) 'Controlling government spending and deficits: trends in the 1980s and prospects in the 1990s.' *OECD Economic Studies* No. 17.

Packman, J. (1975) *The Child's Generation: Child Care Policy from Curtis to Houghton*. Oxford: Blackwell; London: Martin Robertson.

Padgett, S. and Paterson, W.E. (1991) *A History of Social Democracy in Postwar Europe*. Harlow: Longman.

Page, R.M. (1991) 'Social welfare since the war' in Crafts, N.F.R. and Woodward, N. (eds) *The British Economy Since 1945*. Oxford: Clarendon Press.

Papadakis, E. and Taylor-Gooby, P. (1987) *The Private Provision of Public Welfare*. Brighton: Wheatsheaf.

Parker, H. (1989) *Instead of the Dole*. London: Routledge.

Parker, R.A. (1970) 'The future of the personal social services' in Robson, W.A. and Crick, B. (eds) *The Future of the Social Services*. London: Penguin Books.

Parry, R. (1991) 'The privatisation of welfare under the Thatcher government.' *Business in the Contemporary World*, Spring.

Parsons, W. (1982) 'Politics without promises: the crisis of overload and governability.' *Parliamentary Affairs* 35(4): 421–35.

Paton, C. (1990) 'The Prime Minister's review of the National Health Service and the 1989 White Paper Working for Patients' in Manning, N. and Ungerson, C. (eds) *Social Policy Review 1989–90*. London: Longman.

Patten, J. (1992) 'The future of education.' *Independent*, 24 April.

Pearce, B. and Wilcox, S. (1991) *Home-Ownership, Taxation and the Economy: The Economic and Social Effects of the Abolition of Mortgage Interest Tax Relief*. York: Joseph Rowntree Foundation.

Pfaller, A., Gough, I. and Therborn, G. (1991) *Can the Welfare State Compete?* Basingstoke: Macmillan.

Phillipson, C. (1992) 'Challenging the spectre of old age: community care for older people in the 1990s' in Manning, N. and Page, R. (eds) *Social Policy Review 4*. Canterbury: The Social Policy Association.

Piachaud, D. (1990) *Poverty and Social Security*. Paper presented at

Suntory-Toyota Seminar on Issues in Social Policy, London School of Economics.

Plowden, B. (1967) 'Children and their Primary Schools', in Maclure, S. (ed. 1986) *Educational Documents*. London: Methuen.

Powell, E. (1966) *Medicine and Politics*. London: Pitman.

—— (1970) *Income Tax at 4/3 in the £*. London: Tom Stacey.

Prime, R. (1987) *Developing Services for Black and Ethnic Minority Elders in London: Overview and Action Plan*. Social Services Inspectorate, DoH. London: HMSO.

Prime Minister's Office (1991) *The Citizen's Charter: Raising the Standard*, Cm 1599. London: HMSO.

Pym, F. (1985) *The Politics of Consent*. London: Sphere Books.

Reinhardt, U.E. (1990) 'Respondent' in *Health Care Systems in Transition: The Search for Efficiency*. OECD Social Policy Studies No.7. Paris: OECD: 105–12.

Riddell, P. (1991) *The Thatcher Era and its Legacy*. Oxford: Blackwell.

Robbins, Lord (1963) *Report of the Committee on Higher Education* in Maclure, S. (ed. 1986) *Educational Documents*. London: Methuen.

Robinson, R. (1986) 'Restructuring the welfare state: an analysis of public expenditure, 1979/80–1984/5.' *Journal of Social Policy* 15: 1–22.

Robinson, R. and Judge, K. (1987) *Public Expenditure and the NHS: Trends and Prospects*. London: King's Fund Institute.

Rogow, A. and Shore, P. (1955) *The Labour Government and British Industry, 1945–1951*. Oxford: Blackwell.

Roll, J. (1991) 'One in ten: lone parent families in the European Community' in Manning, N. (ed.) *Social Policy Review, 1990–91*. London: Longman.

Room, G. (1991) 'A time for change' in Becker, S. (ed.) *Windows of Opportunity: Public Policy and the Poor*. London: Child Poverty Action Group.

Room, G., Lawson, R. and Laczko, F. (1989) ' "New Poverty" in the European Community.' *Policy and Politics* 17 (2).

Rose, R. and Peters, G. (1979) *Can Governments Go Bankrupt?* Basingstoke: Macmillan.

Royal Commission on the Distribution of Income and Wealth (1979) *Report*. London: HMSO.

Royal National Institute for the Blind (RNIB) (1991) *Blind and Partially Sighted Adults in the UK*. London: RNIB.

Salter, B. (1992) *Policy Paradox and the Rationing Issue: Managing the Tensions*. Canterbury: Centre for Health Services Studies, University of Kent.

Saunders, P. and Harris, C. (n.d.) *Popular Attitudes to State Welfare Services: A Growing Demand for Alternatives?* Research Report 11. London: Social Affairs Unit.

Saunders, P. and Klau, F. (1985) 'The role of the public sector.' *OECD Economic Studies* 4.

Schorr, A.L. (1992) *The Personal Social Services: An Outside View*. York: Joseph Rowntree Foundation.

Seebohm Committee (1968) *Report of the Committee on Local Authority and Allied Personal Social Services*, Cm 3703. London: HMSO.

Seldon, A. (1977) *Charge!* London: Temple-Smith.
—— (1981) *Wither the Welfare State?* London: Institute of Economic Affairs.
Sharpe, L.J. and Newton, K. (1984) *Does Politics Matter? The Determinants of Public Policy.* Oxford: Clarendon Press.
Silburn, R. (1992) 'The changing landscape of poverty' in Manning, N. and Page, R. (eds) *Social Policy Review 4.* Canterbury: Social Policy Association: 134–53.
Smith, D. (1987) *The Rise and Fall of Monetarism.* London: Penguin.
—— (1989) *North and South: Britain's Economic, Social and Political Divide.* London: Penguin.
Smith, J.G. (1992) *Full Employment in the 1990s.* London: Institute of Public Policy Research.
Smithers, R. (1991) 'Record 44,000 owners give up homes.' *Guardian,* 15 February.
Social and Liberal Democrats (SLD) (1989a) *Common Benefit,* Federal Green Paper No.11. London: SLD.
—— (1989b) *Housing: A Time for Action,* English White Paper No.2. Hebden Bridge: Hebden Royd Publications.
—— (1989c) *Prescription for Health.* London: SLD.
Social Security Select Committee (SSSC) (1991a) *Low Income Statistics: Households Below Average Income Tables 1989,* House of Commons Papers Session 1988–9 No.437–i. London: HMSO.
—— (1991b) *The Organisation and Administration of the Department of Social Security – Minutes of Evidence,* House of Commons Papers Session 1990–1 No.550–ii and 1991–2 No.19–i. London: HMSO.
—— (1992) *The Operation of Pension Funds,* House of Commons Papers Session 1991–2 No.61–II. London: HMSO.
Spence, A. (1990) 'Labour force outlook to 2001.' *Employment Gazette* 98(4), April: 186–98.
Stevens, B. (1992) 'Prospects for privatisation in OECD countries.' *National Westminster Quarterly Review,* August, 2–22.
Taylor-Gooby, P. (1985) *Public Opinion, Ideology and State Welfare.* London: Routledge & Kegan Paul.
—— (1987) 'Citizenship and welfare' in Jowell, R., Witherspoon, S. and Brooks, L. (eds) *British Social Attitudes, 1987.* London: Gower.
—— (1990) 'Social welfare: the unkindest cuts' in Jowell *et al.* (eds) *British Social Attitudes: The Seventh Report.* Aldershot: Gower.
—— (1991) *Social Change, Social Welfare and Social Science.* London: Harvester Wheatsheaf.
Taylor-Gooby, P. and Lawson, R. (1992) *Markets and Managers: New Directions in Welfare Policy.* Milton Keynes: Open University Press.
Thain, C. and Wright, M. (1990) 'Coping with difficulty: The Treasury and public expenditure, 1976–1989.' *Policy and Politics* 18: 1–16.
Thane, P. (1982) *The Foundations of the Welfare State.* Harlow: Longman.
Thatcher, M. (1989) *The Revival of Britain: Speeches on Home and European Affairs 1975–1988,* compiled by A.B. Cooke. London: Aurum Press.
Titmuss, R. (1955) 'Pension systems and population change.' *Political Quarterly* 26: 152–66.

—— (1962) *Income Distribution and Social Change*. London: Allen & Unwin.

—— (1968) *Commitment to Welfare*. London: Allen & Unwin.

—— (1971) 'Welfare rights, law and discretion.' *Political Quarterly* 42 (2).

Townsend, P. (1958) 'A society for people' in Mackenzie, N. (ed.) *Conviction*. London: MacGibbon & Kee.

—— (1991) *The Poor are Poorer*. Statistical Monitoring Unit, University of Bristol.

—— (1992) *Hard Times: the Prospects for European Social Policy*. Eleanor Rathbone Memorial Lecture. Liverpool: Liverpool University Press.

UCCA (1990) *Statistical Supplement to the 27th Report, 1988–9*. London: UCCA.

Utting Report (1991) *Children in the Public Care: A Review of Residential Care*. London: HMSO.

Walden, G. (1992) 'Home-ownership, a fetish we can well do without.' *Daily Telegraph*, 20 July.

Walker, A. and Walker, C. (eds) (1987) *The Growing Divide*. London: Child Poverty Action Group.

Wicks, M. (1987) *A Future for All*. Harmondsworth: Penguin.

—— (1990) 'The battle for the family.' *Marxism Today*, August: 28–32.

Widdowson, B. (1987) 'Homelessness in the International Year of Shelter for the Homeless' in Brenton, M. and Ungerson, C. (eds) *Year Book of Social Policy 1986–87*. Harlow: Longman.

Williams, F. (1989) *Social Policy: A Critical Introduction*. Oxford: Polity Press.

Williams, S.J., Calnan, M. and Cant, S. (1991) 'Health promotion and disease prevention in the 1990s.' *Medical Sociology News* 16 (3): 20–9.

Wistow, G. and Henwood, M. (1991) 'Caring for people: elegant model or flawed design?' in Manning, N. (ed.) *Social Policy Review 1990–91*. London: Longman.

Worswick, G.D.N. (1991) *Unemployment: A Problem of Policy. An Analysis of British Experience and Prospects*. Cambridge: Cambridge University Press.

Young, D. (1985) *Enterprise Regained*. London: Conservative Party.

—— (1986) *Enterprises*, Stockton Lecture. London: London Business School.

Index